# TRANSFERENCE-FOCUSED PSYCHOTHERAPY
## FOR ADOLESCENTS WITH
# SEVERE PERSONALITY DISORDERS

# TRANSFERENCE-FOCUSED PSYCHOTHERAPY
## FOR ADOLESCENTS WITH
# SEVERE PERSONALITY DISORDERS

Lina Normandin, Ph.D.

Karin Ensink, Ph.D.

Alan Weiner, Ph.D.

Otto F. Kernberg, M.D.

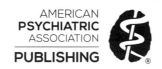

AMERICAN
PSYCHIATRIC
ASSOCIATION
PUBLISHING

If you wish to buy 50 or more copies of the same title, please go to www.appi.org/special-discounts for more information.

First Edition

Manufactured in the United States of America on acid-free paper
25   24   23   22   21      5   4   3   2   1

American Psychiatric Association Publishing
800 Maine Avenue SW, Suite 900
Washington, DC 20024-2812
www.appi.org

**Library of Congress Cataloging-in-Publication Data**
Names: Normandin, Lina, author. | Ensink, Karin, author. | Weiner, Alan, author. | Kernberg, Otto F., author. | American Psychiatric Association, publisher.
Title: Transference-focused psychotherapy for adolescents with severe personality disorders / Lina Normandin, Karin Ensink, Alan Weiner, Otto F. Kernberg.
Description: First edition. | Washington, DC : American Psychiatric Association Publishing, [2021] | Includes bibliographical references and index.
Identifiers: LCCN 2021005934 (print) | LCCN 2021005935 (ebook) | ISBN 9781615373147 (paperback) | ISBN 9781615373543 (ebook)
Subjects: MESH: Personality Disorders—therapy | Adolescent | Psychotherapy, Psychodynamic—methods | Transference, Psychology
Classification: LCC RC554 (print) | LCC RC554 (ebook) | NLM WS 470.P3 | DDC 616.85/81—dc23
LC record available at https://lccn.loc.gov/2021005934
LC ebook record available at https://lccn.loc.gov/2021005935

**British Library Cataloguing in Publication Data**
A CIP record is available from the British Library.

This book is dedicated to our children and grandchildren, as well as our teacher, Paulina Kernberg, who started this journey of helping adolescents with personality disorders. It is also dedicated to our adolescent patients who convinced us that young people with personality disorders deserve specialized treatments as well as therapists who expect the best from them.

# Contents

# PART I

## Models of Psychopathology and Normal Development for Understanding Personality Disorders at Adolescence

# PART II

## Therapeutic Approach

# PART III

### Processes and Applications

# APPENDIX

# About the Authors

**Lina Normandin, Ph.D.,** is professor of psychology at Université Laval in Quebec, Canada, and researcher at and director of the Child and Adolescent Research and Treatment Unit at the Université Laval Outpatient Clinic.

**Karin Ensink, Ph.D.,** is professor of psychology at Université Laval in Quebec, Canada, and principal researcher at the Child and Adolescent Research and Treatment Unit at the Université Laval Outpatient Clinic.

**Alan Weiner, Ph.D.,** is a voluntary faculty member of Weill Cornell Medical College Department of Psychiatry, where he supervises advanced students in psychiatry and psychology, and a consultant in the Division of Child and Adolescent Psychiatry at Payne Whitney Westchester.

**Otto F. Kernberg, M.D.,** is director of the Personality Disorders Institute at Weill Cornell Medical College, professor of psychiatry at Weill Cornell Medical College, and training and supervising analyst at the Columbia University Center for Psychoanalytic Training and Research in New York, New York.

# Preface

**UNDER OPTIMAL** circumstances, adolescence is an exhilarating time of life, a period of personal expansion into new territories of knowledge and skills, interests and dreams, that prepares the adolescent for mature engagement and satisfaction in work, love, and play. It is the gateway to biological and psychological enjoyment of adult love, sexuality, and consolidation of lifelong friendships and social networks. Adolescence is a time for entering the currents of history and culture, and taking one's own place in nature and society.

However, this developmental period is not without its challenges. Painful recognition of the inevitability and prevalence of human aggression, rivalry, competition, envy, betrayal, and one's own limitations signals the end of infantile naivete. It is a time for learning to maintain faith, love, confidence, and trust in the context of disappointments, ambiguity, and disillusionment. With optimal psychological resources and external supports, meeting the challenge of these adversities forges sufficient resilience to weather the storms. But, with a troubled developmental history and a traumatizing and restrictive personal and social environment, adolescent growth and expansion may be severely curtailed and distorted. Growing resentment over a world that seems hostile and indifferent, where all roads to personal expansion are blocked, and the attainment of a stable identity undermined by insecurity and loneliness combine to put the overall well-being and mental health of the adolescent at a severe disadvantage.

Transference-Focused Psychotherapy for Adolescents (TFP-A) is a specialized psychodynamic psychotherapy geared toward exploring and resolving the conflicts linked to negative experience and the behaviors that express severe threats to and limitations of normal adolescent development. TFP-A is a clinically and empirically tested application of psychoanalytic theory and technique to the specific disturbances of identity that signal the development of a severe personality disorder. The description of this treatment is the fundamental objective of this manual. While the techniques employed pay close attention to the patient's current dilemmas and symptoms, our ultimate objective is to resolve the intrapsychic restrictions that interfere with the adolescent's normal development in the age-appropriate realms of love, sexuality, friendship, intimacy, and pursuit of educational and creative success. In the process, the adolescent's capacity for both autonomous and independent functioning, and a more mature and collaborative engagement with the family of origin, are part of the intended growth of his or her social functioning.

The analytically oriented psychotherapist needs to be alert to the complexity and challenges to establishing adolescent identity and open to the uncertainties of new experiences and to the fearful withdrawal from what threatens to reopen traumatic experiences from the past. The therapist needs to empathize with the nonconventional presentation of the patient while holding in mind the realistic tasks that need to be assumed by the adolescent. The qualities of flexibility and firmness, and tolerance and understanding for aberrant values and modes of relating, will facilitate the integration of the patient's internal experience. The therapist needs to confront the adolescent with his or her wide horizon of potential growth and success, and harbor an implicit ideal vision of what he or she might achieve, while respecting the reality of the concrete treatment situation. Ideally, the therapist represents a "third voice," an interpreter and mediator between the adolescent, the parent(s), and conventional society and its values. The ultimate goal is to foster ego integration sufficient to allow the adolescent to proceed under his or her own agency.

# Introduction and Overview of the Manual

**THE PREVALENCE** of borderline personality disorder (BPD) is estimated at around 11% among adolescents (Chanen et al. 2004; Feenstra et al. 2011), rising to 22% among young people ages 15–25 (Chanen and McCutcheon 2008), and 49% in hospitalized adolescents (Grilo et al. 1996). Within other personality disorder (PD) categories, the prevalence rates range from 10% to 15% within this age group (Feenstra et al. 2011; Johnson et al. 2005). Longitudinal data show a normative increase in BPD traits after puberty, with prevalence of the disorder reaching its peak in early adulthood and subsequently declining over subsequent decades (Chanen and Kaess 2012; Cohen et al. 2005; Shiner 2009; Tackett et al. 2009). Its manifestations are mostly marked mood swings, affective instability, and aggression and impulsivity, including self-harm, suicide attempts, and substance abuse. There is irrefutable evidence that PD diagnoses in adolescents have validity and stability over time (Chanen and Kaess 2012; Cohen et al. 2005; Sharp and Fonagy 2015).

Despite converging evidence that PDs emerge in childhood and are clearly evident in adolescence, clinicians have remained reluctant to diagnose PDs before age 18. This reluctance is partly due to concerns that behaviors that might be normative in children and adolescents, and part of normal adolescent sturm und drang, might be misdiagnosed as signs of BPD and that diagnosis may lead to unnecessary stigmatization. The advocacy work of pioneers like Paulina Kernberg (1997; Kernberg et al. 2000; Terr and Kernberg 1990) and research over the past decade (Chanen and Kaess 2012; Chanen and McCutcheon 2008; Miller et al. 2008) have done much to dispel these concerns, and it is evident that a constellation of PD-type symptoms can be observed in children and adolescents. Furthermore, it is evident that personality difficulties are unlikely to resolve without specific interventions that are developed explicitly to treat adolescents with PDs.

Stigmatization of adolescents with PDs remains a real concern, and much remains to be done to address this through education and training of mental health staff to understand and respond to adolescents with PDs, as well as through making available treatments designed to address the challenges adolescents and young people afflicted with personality difficulties pose to others and experience themselves. The hesitation of clinicians to diagnose PDs may have delayed the development of treatment models for this age group. Currently, there is relatively little research on effective treatments for adolescents with PDs. Therefore, we are trying to take up this imperative need for treatment models focusing on adolescent PDs that would have both strong theoretical foundations and manualized interventions.

This manual presents Transference-Focused Psychotherapy for Adolescents (TFP-A), a treatment for adolescents and young people who suffer from severe PDs. It is an adaptation of Transference-Focused Psychotherapy (TFP) for adults suffering from BPD (Clarkin et al. 2006; Yeomans et al. 2015). It is grounded in a psychoanalytic object relations approach developed by Otto Kernberg (1984, 1993), as well as developmental theory and empirical research (Clarkin and Posner 2005; Clarkin et al. 2007; Doering et al. 2010; Levy 2005; Levy et al. 1999). In this treatment, PD is seen as a disturbance in the process of identity formation. Adolescence, which is the pivotal developmental period for identity formation and personality consolidation (Erikson 1968), is therefore seen as a sensitive period to intervene.

This manual is inspired by Paulina Kernberg's exceptional work with children and adolescents. She was the director of the Residency Program in Child and Adolescent Psychiatry at the New York Presbyterian Hospital, Payne Whitney Westchester–Weill Cornell Medical Center from 1978 until she died in 2006. She was also a teacher, supervisor, and training analyst at the Columbia University Center for Psychoanalytic Training and Research. She was probably the first to draw attention to and write about early manifestations and development of PDs, including borderline and narcissistic PDs in children (Kernberg et al. 1998; Terr and Kernberg 1990). She elucidated assessment criteria and treatment approaches for a wide spectrum of PDs observed in children and adolescents, and she developed assessment interviews to measure the level of personality integration in adolescents. Several aspects of her thinking are reflected in this manual.

# Features and Goals of TFP-A

The specificity of TFP-A includes a focus on facilitating identity integration and personality consolidation through 1) addressing dominant pathological object relations as they are activated and manifested in the here-and-now interactions with the therapist; 2) elaborating on a contract with adolescents to help them reduce, contain, and ultimately control acting out while stimulating curiosity about their motivations and prioritizing mentalizing about self and others as well as about the consequences of their actions and their future; 3) offering a specific approach to supporting parents, facilitating their collaboration, and reducing their interference as well as creating a mental space for adolescents where they can develop autonomy and gradually assume responsibility for their difficulties[1]; and 4) placing an emphasis on interpreting transference and countertransference reactions in order to identify split self and other representations that are viewed as an impediment to the flow of the developmental processes and undermine personality consolidation, as well as the adaptive use of acquired mentalization capacities in order to deal with the challenges of adolescence and the future.

TFP-A is also grounded in an understanding of the major structural changes and developmental tasks that the adolescent is facing. Therefore, the aim of TFP-A is to scaffold structural changes and oversee developmental challenges central to adolescence while addressing pathology in object relations and identity integration that disrupts these developments. The major structural changes concern constituents of personality (self-image, ideal self, and self-esteem as well as moral and ethics, sexuality and eroticism, concern, and reparation wishes) that have to be consolidated. The developmental challenges include becoming more independent from family, establishing their own social networks, negotiating sexual relationships, and forming romantic and couple relationships, while clarifying future life and career goals and pursuing these purposefully. In contexts of family dysfunction or disorganization, parental mental illness, substance abuse, and violence or when there is little family support, adolescents without personality pathology may also have difficulties successfully engaging with the challenges of adolescence, but they are generally receptive and responsive to help when help is offered. When clinicians are attempting to distinguish and identify personality pathology, it is important for them to consider the developmental history of adolescent patients as well as their current functioning with family and peers, at school or work, while also being well informed

---

[1]In essence, the work with parents supports them in their use of authority when appropriate and when adolescents are potentially in danger, but also helps the parents to step back to facilitate separation and individuation and to decrease conflict, overt aggression, and battles over power and control that can derail therapeutic work and progress

regarding developmental issues and structural changes specific to adolescence. This provides a framework that facilitates understanding the adolescent's developing sense of self and others—the process of identity formation—as it unfolds during separation from family and entry into the adult world. Radical failures in engaging with the normative challenges of adolescence and the manifestation of immature internal structures are features of adolescent PDs.

# Organization of the Manual

In Part I of the manual, we first explore the phenomenology of PDs, examine the validity of PD as a diagnostic category at adolescence, and review the etiological risk factors for its development. We then present an understanding of PDs grounded in Otto Kernberg's contemporary object relations theory and the notion of "identity diffusion," which is an incapacity to convey to an observer an integrated description of self and the equal lack of capacity to convey an integrated view of significant others (Kernberg 2012). Identity diffusion is hypothesized to result from the dominance of severe aggressive impulses, whether genetically determined, resulting from a temperamentally established predominance of negative affects or lack of cognitive control and contextualization of affects, or following severely pathological attachment or traumatic experiences in early infancy and childhood. We follow this discussion with a presentation of major structural changes and developmental tasks that typically developing adolescents are encountering. It is hypothesized that identity diffusion puts significant pressure on the normal maturational processes that are geared toward separation and individuation: the attainment of a realistic self-image, self-esteem, and self-ideal; the completion of an integrated system of morality and ethical values; the fulfillment of sexual and romantic intimacy; friendship and commitments; the effectiveness and gratification in school or work or in choosing a career; and the actualization of personal creativity—all of which are, in whole or in part, consolidated at adolescence. These two levels of analysis serve to propose an integrated conception of the pathology of PDs and its interferences on normal development that will become the main targets of TFP-A. It is our belief that to be effective in treating PDs at adolescence, a therapist must keep in mind a model of the PD pathology and a model of normal development in order to be sensitive to what is typical and what is atypical in the adolescent's behaviors and relationships, as well as to "preview" and to "focus on" imminent maturational trends, structural changes, and developmental challenges ahead.

In Part II, we present the therapeutic approach used in TFP-A. The main goal of the treatment is identity integration and personality consolidation. We consider that the integration of mutually split-off idealized and persecutory internalized object relations that surface in the transference enables the adolescent to achieve a coherent, realistic, and stable experience of self and others that equips him or her to face developmental challenges and that is consolidated in specific structures of the personality. We consider that by addressing such disabling difficulties in the personality structure, the adolescent may resume the normal course of personality development sufficiently to engage in studies/work and make choices regarding his or her future work and develop the capacity to have meaningful interpersonal and romantic relationships. To achieve this goal, we propose a series of steps, so-called strategies of TFP-A, involving attempts to integrate part-self and part-object representations through a process in which underlying representations are recognized and marked by the therapist and then delineated as characteristic patterns of experiencing, relating, or disrupting developmental challenges. Part II of this manual (Chapter 4) also focuses on assessment to clarify diagnosis, the presence of a PD, the critical areas of dysfunction, and the level of personality organization as distinct from the identity crisis of normal adolescence. Typically, adolescents and their parents do not present for therapy saying that they think they may have a PD, although there is a somewhat greater awareness of borderline and narcissistic PDs than in the past. Instead, they describe concerns about anxiety, mood, anger, or interpersonal functioning with family, peers, and school. The clinician, in turn, explains the assessment process to the adolescent and parents. This discussion focuses on the purpose of assessment, including the need to understand the nature of the adolescent's problems, culminating in a determination of an appropriate treatment choice. Both the adolescent and the parents are involved in this process.

Chapter 5 in Part II describes the establishment of a treatment contract, considered the first of a series of TFP-A tactics. This phase consists of negotiating a verbal treatment contract implicating the adolescent, the parents, and the therapist and precedes the start of the therapy. The specific techniques of TFP-A—the moment-to-moment interventions the therapist engages in with the patient in therapy sessions—are then described in Chapter 6. We present six basic techniques at the core of TFP-A: the active stance of the therapist, the interpretative process, the analysis of transference, the analysis of countertransference, technical neutrality, and developmentally informed interventions. We then outline, in Chapter 7, tactics that the therapist uses to maintain the treatment frame, attend to parental concerns, clarify involvement, maintain the focus on developing the adolescent's internal resources rather than to manage behaviors, identify priority themes, manage adolescent resistances and negative therapeutic reactions, and "preview" developmental and structural changes ahead.

In Part III, we present how TFP-A unfolds across different phases of the treatment. We include the TFP-A Manual Adherence and Competence Scale as an appendix.

# PART I

Models of Psychopathology and Normal Development for Understanding Personality Disorders at Adolescence

# CHAPTER 1

# Personality Disorders at Adolescence

## Phenomenology, Development, and Construct Validity

**IN THIS CHAPTER,** we outline the phenomenology and research regarding personality disorders (PDs) in adolescents and young people and discuss how to recognize some of the ways in which PDs present. We then present a developmental model of borderline personality disorder (BPD) in adolescence, describing how BPD develops, what the risk factors are, and why BPD appears to become particularly evident in adolescence. In Chapter 2, we will propose a definition of personality and outline its normal development and contrast this with personality pathology.

## Phenomenology and Diagnosis of Personality Disorders at Adolescence

Already by the late 1990s Paulina Kernberg (1997; Kernberg et al. 2000) had identified a constellation of severe symptoms indicative of PDs in adolescents. This led her to advocate for awareness of adolescent BPD. She argued that it is important to diagnose BPD in young people and that early intervention is essential to help adolescents address the severe disruptions associated with BPD and reduce the negative impacts during this critical period so as to help adolescents resume a more adaptive course of development. Current guidelines published by the U.K. National Institute for Health and Care Excellence (NICE) (National Institute for Clinical Excellence 2009; see also Kendall et al. 2009) and the Australian National Health and Medical Research Council (2012) also provide clear support for diagnosing BPD in young people, and they propose a less restrictive age range than DSM-5 and ICD-10. The World Health Organization (WHO) Guideline Development Group (GDG; World Health Organization 2009) also indicates that their proposals about BPD apply to young people postpubertally. Furthermore, they stipulate that in some circumstances the diagnosis of BPD may be warranted even before age 13. The GDG recommends that clinical features such as suicidal/self-harming behaviors, significant emotional instability, increasing intensity of symptoms, multiple comorbidities, poor response to ongoing treatment, and high level of functional impairment should alert clinicians to assess for the possibility of BPD as part of a comprehensive clinical evaluation.

Despite these practice guidelines clearly indicating that adult criteria can be reliably used for diagnosing and treating young people from age 14 on, clinicians remain hesitant to diagnose BPD in adolescents or young adults. Surveys show that less than 40% of clinicians who work with adolescents diagnose BPD in patients younger than 18 years (Griffiths 2011; Laurenssen et al. 2013). Common concerns clinicians give for not wanting to make the diagnosis are that the problems may be transient (41%); that DSM-IV-TR does not allow PD diagnoses in adolescents (26%); and that the diagnosis could be stigmatizing (9%). In sum, these findings suggest that scientific findings and practice guidelines are not currently being applied and integrated into clinical practice (Coghill 2014).

BPD in young people is also frequently overlooked because of its comorbidity with mood disorders (i.e., anxiety, depression, and bipolar disorders) and behavior difficulties (e.g., oppositional defiant disorder [ODD], conduct disorder [CD]). When mood and behavior difficulties are present, there is a tendency to overlook the possibility of PD and focus only on Axis I disorders. However, considering that untreated BPD in adolescence predicts Axis I and II problems in adulthood (Cohen et al. 2007), it is important for clinicians to be alert to BPD features in adolescents and preadolescents. Identifying and treating BPD is essential to lessen the likelihood of undiagnosed and untreated BPD disrupting the course of development, undermining successful engagement with key developmental challenges, and increasing the risk of maladjustment and psychopathology in adulthood.

# DSM-5 Criteria and Relevant Research

There has been an upsurge in interest in BPD in adolescents in light of evidence that it can be reliably diagnosed (Glenn and Klonsky 2013; Michonski et al. 2013), affects a sizable percentage of adolescents (Miller et al. 2008), and is associated with marked dysfunction in terms of self and interpersonal functioning (Glenn and Klonsky 2013; Winsper et al. 2015). Studies show that 33% of adolescent inpatients (Ha et al. 2014) and 22% of adolescent outpatients (Chanen and McCutcheon 2013) have presentations that meet criteria for BPD. The prevalence of BPD in adolescents appears to be at least as high, if not higher, than in adulthood (Chabrol et al. 2001; Cohen et al. 2005; Johnson et al. 2006; Lewinsohn et al. 1997). Furthermore, BPD affects a relatively high percentage of adolescents in the community, with some studies indicating that as many as 14.6% of 14-year-olds and 12.7% of 16-year-olds have symptoms that meet criteria for BPD (Johnson et al. 2008). In sum, there is convincing evidence that BPD is identifiable in adolescence and is distinguishable from "normal adolescence" (Bornovalova et al. 2009; DeFife et al. 2013; Hutsebaut et al. 2013; Sharp and Fonagy 2015; Shiner 2005; Westen et al. 2014). In fact, research suggests that storminess and turmoil is relatively rare and that most adolescents engage with the transition to adulthood and the physical and other changes with surprisingly little upheaval (Cicchetti and Rogosch 2002).

DSM-5 currently includes a mixed categorical and dimensional approach to the diagnosis of BPD (Oldham 2018; Skodol 2018; Skodol et al. 2014), with a categorical approach outlined in Section II and a dimensional approach described in Section III. This hybrid model is the outcome of an attempt to replace the categorical approach with a dimensional one more consistent with empirical evidence suggesting that BPD is best considered as levels of disturbance across a range of different functional domains. However, concerns that this dimensional approach may have disadvantages in clinical settings, where clinicians tend to rely on a categorical approach to diagnose and organize interventions, led to the retention of the categorical diagnostic criteria. At present, Section II responds to the needs of clinicians who are used to thinking categorically, while Section III provides an alternative dimensional approach. Although the Section III approach may be more compatible with research and thinking about the processes underlying the pathology, its practical utility in real-life clinical settings remains to be seen. Section II specifies that the diagnosis of PD can be applied to children and adolescents "in those relatively unusual instances in which the individual's particular maladaptive personality traits appear to be pervasive, persistent, and unlikely to be limited to a particular developmental stage or another mental disorder" (American Psychiatric Association 2013, p. 647). Furthermore, a duration of only 1 year is necessary for the diagnosis of child and adolescent PD, in contrast to the 2 years required before adult BPD can be diagnosed.

The criteria specified in Section II of DSM-5 for the diagnosis of BPD include abandonment fears, unstable and intense interpersonal relationships, identity disturbance, impulsivity, suicidal behaviors, affective instability, chronic feelings of emptiness, inappropriate intense anger, and transient stress-related paranoid ideation or severe dissociative symptoms. BPD can be clearly and systematically distinguished from externalizing and internalizing pathology by the presence of a mix of both internalizing and externalizing symptoms. Furthermore, the symptoms of BPD in terms of their pervasiveness and severity are clearly distinguishable from the range of reactions and "ups and downs" that adolescents may have over the course of engaging with the characteristic challenges, inevitable frustrations, and possible failures of this period.

As a complement to Section II, Section III of DSM-5 provides a dimensional approach. A standard template is provided in Section III that requires clinicians to consider functioning in terms of two criteria. Criterion A requires evaluation of difficulties involving identity, self-direction, empathy, and intimacy. Criterion B requires the presence of at least four of the following seven traits of personality pathology: emotional lability, anxiousness, separation insecurity, depressivity, impulsivity, risk taking, and hostility. Any PD must meet two primary defining criteria: Criterion A (moderate or greater impairment in personality functioning in the realms of self [identity and self-direction] and interpersonal relationships [empathy and intimacy]) and Criterion B (presence of one or more pathological personality traits in any of five trait domains [negative affectivity, detachment, antagonism, disinhibition, and psychoticism]). Criteria C through G must also be satisfied, as in DSM-5 Section II: Criterion C (inflexibility and pervasiveness), Criterion D (relatively stable impairment in functioning over time), Criterion E (impairment not better explained by another mental disorder), Criterion F (impairment not solely attributable to substance use or a medical condition), and Criterion G (impairment not better understood as a normal developmental stage or a normal aspect of a sociocultural environment).

# Borderline Personality Disorder: A Disorder Encompassing Heterogeneous Symptoms

Considering the fact that BPD criteria can be met by individuals with very different symptom combinations, questions have been raised regarding the validity and phenomenology of BPD and whether the DSM criteria describe a single disorder. Current evidence based on studies of BPD in adolescents (Michonski 2014) suggests that while multidimensional models best describe the phenomena of BPD, a unidimensional model is also supported, and the dimensions or factors hang together and are strongly related, consistent with the notion of BPD as a unidimensional construct and disorder (Michonski 2014; Sharp and Fonagy 2015). From a scientific/research perspective, further studies are required to examine whether BPD in adolescents can be demonstrated to be unidimensional and differentiated from other PDs, or whether, as in adults, it is difficult to demonstrate undimensionality for BPD when PDs are analyzed simultaneously.

Another important line of investigation has examined whether particular symptoms can be identified that are most predictive of adolescent BPD. Earlier studies identified chronic feelings of emptiness and inappropriate intense anger (Garnet et al. 1994), and later studies pointed to identity disturbance, affective liability, and inappropriate intense anger (Becker et al. 2002; McManus et al. 1984; Meijer et al. 1998; Westen et al. 2011) as most predictive of adolescent BPD. Furthermore, there appears to be gender-related differences in predictors of BPD, with paranoid ideation in boys and identity disturbance in girls appearing most predictive (Michonski et al. 2013). BPD frequently is comorbid with internalizing and externalizing disorders, with comorbidity rates ranging from 70.6% to 86% in adolescent clinical samples (Ha et al. 2014; Speranza et al. 2011). This suggests that BPD represents a confluence of internalizing and externalizing disorders that is best understood in terms of a separate disorder (Sharp and Fonagy 2015).

In line with the suggestion that BPD represents a confluence of internalizing and externalizing disorders, BPD in adolescents has been shown to be one of the best predictors of subsequent self-harm (Bégin et al. 2017; Glenn and Klonsky 2011; Wilcox et al. 2012) and suicidality (Yen et al. 2013). Adolescent BPD is also associated with an increased risk of sexual risk taking and sexually transmitted diseases (Chanen et al. 2007). Adolescents with BPD are at particularly elevated risk of manifesting impairments in academic and social functioning, and longitudinal studies show that these impairments in functioning persist into adulthood (Crawford et al. 2008; Gunderson et al. 2011; Winograd et al. 2008; Zanarini et al. 2006), although individual symptoms may change.

Table 1–1 presents core diagnostic features identified for BPD in adolescents (from Fossati 2014), early childhood markers of vulnerability to BPD, and positive outcome ("resilience") factors. In the case that follows, we present a typical manifestation of an adolescent with BPD.

# Case 1: Amanda

Amanda, a 16-year-old, was admitted to an inpatient psychiatric unit because she made a suicide attempt after her boyfriend ended their relationship. The relationship was intense and stormy, with Amanda becoming distraught and physically violent when her boyfriend as much as talked to other girls at school or whenever he made plans to go out without her to socialize with his friends or pursue his sports. This triggered crises and affect storms during which she oscillated between tearfully clinging to him and expressing intense anxiety and fears of abandonment and angrily accusing him of using her and wanting to get away from her when she needed him and wanting to cheat on her. This culminated in her boyfriend suggesting that they stop seeing each other because he needed time to study, felt that he was losing his friends, and was neglecting his sport practice because he always felt guilty when he left Amanda alone at home. Amanda reacted by saying that she did not want to live without him; she locked herself in the bedroom, engaged in self-harm, posted dramatic threats of suicide on social media, and phoned and texted him incessantly. When he blocked her number, she took an overdose and left a suicide note.

Her parents reported that as a child Amanda displayed intense negative emotional reactions to ordinary disappointments and frustrations. She always seemed unhappy or sad, and quickly became angry and resentful when she felt that others had treated her unfairly; she blamed others for being mean without apparent awareness of her own aggression and how this provoked the reactions she accused others of. She quickly lost her friends because, despite initially being excited and very enthusiastic, she rapidly found fatal flaws in them when they showed interest in other activities or friends, declined her invitations, or seemed less motivated than she was to talk or text with her. Following these times when she ended a friendship after dramatic accusations, she became preoccupied about what she felt was her friends' selfishness or betrayal. She then became demanding of her parents and tearful and resentful when they indicated that they needed to attend to other siblings, even when they spent hours listening to her difficulties and trying to understand and empathize with her

**TABLE 1–1.** Core diagnostic features of borderline personality disorder (BPD) in adolescence, childhood markers of vulnerability to BPD, and positive outcome ("resilience") factors

| | |
|---|---|
| Core diagnostic features | Identity disturbance (particularly for girls) |
| | Inappropriate, intense anger |
| | Paranoid ideation (particularly for boys) |
| | Chronic feelings of emptiness and dissociation proneness |
| Childhood markers of vulnerability | |
| Childhood disorders | Attention-deficit/hyperactivity disorder |
| | Oppositional defiant disorder |
| | Controlling and coercive behaviors toward attachment figures |
| | Poorly defined sense of the self |
| Childhood problem behavior | Hostile, distrustful view of the world |
| | Relational aggression |
| | Intense outbursts of anger |
| | Affective instability |
| Resilience factors | Reflection[a] |
| | Agency[b] |
| | Relatedness[c] |

[a]The capacity and willingness to recognize, experience, and reflect on one's own thoughts, feeling, and motivations.
[b]A sense of oneself as effective and responsible for one's actions.
[c]A valuing relationship that takes the form of openness to the other's perspective and of efforts to engage with others.
*Source.* Fossati 2014.

problems. Furthermore, Amanda did not seem invested in school or sport and seemed to have few interests other than texting and social media; she frequently claimed to be bored at home and gave this as a reason for going out to clubs and bars and coming home late evidently drunk. She spent little time studying, claiming she was too anxious, and was not interested in the material in any case; she frequently claimed to be sick on exam days and was in danger of failing her year. She seemed to have no plans for the future or sense of goals or purposeful action At a recent pool party at the family home, Amanda put on her swimsuit but refused to swim because, as she later confided to her sister, she was ashamed of the cuts she had on her thighs and was afraid that her parents would notice.

# Developmental Precursors and Etiological Risk Factors

The development of BPD is likely a multidetermined process with roots in early childhood that tends to more fully manifest around puberty (Chanen and Kaess 2012; Shiner 2009; Zanarini et al. 2001) and involves complex and interactive biological and psychosocial risk factors (Carlson et al. 2009; Crowell et al. 2009; Lenzenweger and Cicchetti 2005; Paris 2003a, 2003b, 2007). BPD is marked by disturbance in mood (e.g., wide mood swings), impulsivity (e.g., nonsuicidal self-injury, overdoses, substance abuse), and interpersonal dysfunction (e.g., stormy relationship with attachment figures). There is no single explanation for its cause; risk factors vary among patients and reflect the concept of equifinality (Cicchetti and Rogosch 2002), in which different pathways may lead to similar outcomes. Risk factors include *genetic* contributors (Distel et al. 2008), and more specifically inherited biological plasticity genes that interact with positive and negative events (Amad et al. 2014); *temperamental* contributors, which may be noticeable in early infancy and childhood and expressed as negative affectivity, stress reactivity, and impulsivity, which are linked to emotional vulnerability (Goodman et al. 2004; Posner et al. 2003) and which can have a negative impact on others and contribute to the development of poor attachment relations; and *environmental* and *experiential* contributors, such as the manner in which parents interact with, are influenced by, and maintain or modify their child's behaviors, which can also influence gene expression.

## Genetic Risk Factors

There is growing evidence that genetic polymorphisms underlie specific personality traits and that secondary traits (e.g., emotional dysregulation, constraint/conscientiousness) may be sufficient to represent personality pathology (Livesley 2005) as described by some theoretical models. There appears to be a strong heritability component to BPD (Torgersen et al. 2000), with evidence of familial patterns in BPD in which first-degree relatives are more likely to have BPD and BPD symptoms (Zanarini et al. 2005). More specifically, research suggests that genetic factors substantially increase the risk for developing BPD as well as antisocial personality traits, as indexed by examination of the genetics of the serotonin neurotransmitter system (Lyons-Ruth et al. 2007). This genetic effect appears to be independent of the quality of early care. For instance, in a longitudinal study of borderline personality–related characteristics (BPRC;

Belsky et al. 2012), in which twins were examined at ages 7, 10, and 12 years, genetics were found to account for 66% of the variance in BPRC. Variables examined included family history of psychopathology, physical maltreatment, and maternal negative expressed emotion. Furthermore, harsh parental treatment had a more powerful impact on children originating from families with a positive history of the disorder, thereby supporting a diathesis-stress model.

# Temperamental Risk Factors

Extreme temperamental vulnerability may well be one of the most important risk factors for the development of BPD. In a demonstration of the intricate interaction of temperamental and experiential factors, Zanarini and Frankenburg (2007) offered a "complex" model based on more than a decade of empirical research on the etiology of BPD. They suggested that a vulnerable "hyperbolic" temperament is central to the development of BPD. Individuals with this temperament are easily offended, and they work hard to get others to pay attention to their inner pain, often by utilizing indirect means to obtain comfort or support, and will covertly reproach others for their "insensitivity, stupidity, or malevolence." BPD symptoms emerge when these individuals encounter a "kindling" event, which may occur in latency or in early, middle, or late adolescence. Zanarini and Frankenburg (2007) propose that even relatively normative events, such as starting one's first job or beginning one's first intimate relationship, may be stressful enough to be a trigger for these extremely vulnerable individuals.

Rogosch and Cicchetti (2005), while studying the impact of maltreatment in childhood, constructed a BPD precursor composite based on personality, interpersonal relationships, and representational models of the parents, self, and peers, as well as suicidal/self-harming behavior. They found that both maltreatment and attentional control (a particular cognitive dimension of temperament) independently predicted the BPD precursor composite. This finding is consistent with Zanarini and Frankenburg's (2007) model with regard to the interaction of temperament and experience, as well as with Belsky et al.'s (2012) findings, but in addition underscores the importance of considering the contribution of maltreatment experiences.

# Environmental and Experiential Risk Factors

There are a range of findings associating different features of parenting with the development of BPD in children. These features include aspects of early rearing and the quality of caretaking to later interactions and parents' capacity to foster autonomy and promote healthy identity formation.

There is converging evidence that BPD is more likely to develop in children who have experienced neglect and abuse associated with family dysfunction, parental psychopathology, and family interactions that are invalidating, conflictual, negatively critical (Fruzzetti et al. 2005), and unempathic (Guttman and Laporte 2000). Most forms of adversity are more frequently reported by BPD patients, and many of these forms of adversity co-occur (Zanarini et al. 1997, 2000).

Zanarini et al. (2005) reviewed the evidence regarding the link between BPD and maltreatment, including early separation and loss, disturbed parental involvement, experiences of verbal and emotional abuse, experiences of physical and sexual abuse, and experiences of physical and emotional neglect. Prolonged early separations and losses were significantly more common among the childhood histories of BPD patients than among the childhood histories of other diagnostic groups. BPD patients also reported significantly more highly conflictual, distant, or uninvolved relationships with maternal figures. The failure of fathers to be present was another discriminating factor, as were disturbed relationships with both parents. Verbal and emotional abuse was also significantly more present in the histories of patients with BPD than in those of depressed patients or patients with other Axis II pathology. Physical and sexual abuse was also relatively common in the histories of patients with BPD; sexual abuse was significantly more common in patients with BPD than in other psychiatric patient comparison groups, although physical abuse was not. In addition, severity of sexual abuse was related to severity of symptoms. The findings with regard to physical neglect were inconclusive. However, emotional neglect (emotional withdrawal, inconsistent treatment, denial of feelings, lack of a real relationship, parentification of the child, and failure to provide needed protection) was very common among BPD patients and highly discriminating.

As Rogosch and Cicchetti (2005) observed, the similarities in the dysfunctional developmental processes displayed by maltreated children and adult patients with BPD are suggestive of a prospective pathway from childhood maltreatment to BPD. Maltreated children show sequelae across multiple domains of functioning that are similar to the key features of BPD, including affect dysregulation; relationship disturbances with parents and peers; disturbances in representations of self, parents, and peers; cognitive and affective processing anomalies; and maladaptive personality organization (Cicchetti and Valentino 2006). Furthermore, maltreatment is related to suicidal ideation and behavior and psychopathology (Cicchetti and Toth

2016). However, it is important to take into account that although maltreated children are more likely to show precursors of BPD, not all do, and there are also children who have not been abused who display BPD precursors (Rogosch and Cicchetti 2005). Child temperament is likely to interact with and exacerbate parenting vulnerabilities. For example, the home environment is more chaotic for children who are high in extraversion-urgency, but less chaotic for childen with high effortful control (Lemery-Chalfant et al. 2013a, 2013b), likely because children with greater effortful control make fewer demands and provoke less negative caretaking behaviors from more vulnerable parents.

Maltreatment that evokes fear and aggression or involves children being left for long periods without help to regulate affect is known to undermine the development of regulatory processes (Fonagy et al. 2002). Maltreatment may have permanent negative implications for affect regulation through the negative impact of prolonged exposure to high levels of cortisol on the developing hypothalamic-pituitary-adrenal (HPA) axis, with long-term consequences for the physiological processes associated with stress regulation (Cross et al. 2017). Childhood maltreatment has been identified as a risk factor for BPD in adulthood in community samples (Afifi et al. 2011; Widom et al. 2009), as well as in clinical samples (Battle et al. 2004; Chiesa and Fonagy 2014; Sansone et al. 2011). Research on the relationship between maltreatment and BPD in adolescence is more limited, but consistent with the adult literature, there is some evidence that childhood abuse and neglect are risk factors for the development of borderline traits in school-age children and adolescents (Bounoua et al. 2015; Jovev et al. 2013; Zelkowitz et al. 2001). For example, children who experienced sexual abuse were found to be at a fourfold risk of developing borderline personality traits (Zelkowitz et al. 2001). In addition, adolescents who experienced sexual abuse and parental antipathy in combination with others forms of maltreatment were found to manifest significantly more borderline personality features (Bégin et al. 2017).

Theoretical and empirical models suggest an interaction between genetic and environmental factors in the etiology of BPD (Bornovalova et al. 2009; Crowell et al. 2014; Joyce et al. 2003). Consistent with this, maltreatment (physical and psychological abuse) before the age of 10 was found to predict borderline personality traits in 12-year-olds, but genetic vulnerability (measured by psychiatric antecedents in the family) greatly increased the chances that maltreated children would develop borderline personality traits in adolescence (Belsky et al. 2012). In line with this, temperament, which is assumed to be genetically based, has been shown to moderate the expression of borderline pathology in adolescents who experienced abuse and neglect (Jovev et al. 2013).

Lyons-Ruth and colleagues (Khoury et al. 2019; Lyons-Ruth et al. 2013) identified maternal withdrawal and lack of responsiveness as being particularly important in predicting personality disorder and suggested that parental withdrawal may be even more devastating than parental hostility. While this may be a surprising conclusion given previous research highlighting the links between abuse and BPD, it may be that by withdrawing, the parent is failing to comfort the infant when he is distressed, resulting in an escalation rather than regulation of distress and a permanent hyperactivation of the attachment system. This finding may be particularly relevant for understanding the difficulties in affect dysregulation, dependency, and abandonment anxiety commonly experienced by individuals with BPD.

Some studies relevant to understanding etiological factors involve mothers diagnosed with BPD. For instance, mothers who showed deficits in validating their teenager's opinions, were hostile and overpersonalized disagreements, and pushed their teens to agree without attempting to offer satisfying justifications had difficulty supporting their adolescents' autonomy and minimized their children's relatedness (Frankel-Waldheter et al. 2015). They also overpersonalized situations and thereby reduced their child's independent thought and action and attempted to keep them close by using hostile means to inhibit the child's development of relatedness. Mothers with BPD were similar to control mothers in several of their approaches to interacting with their child but showed an increase in role reversal. If, for example, they were expecting their child to satisfy their needs, they could not take on the role of the nurturing parent, especially one who could foster secure attachment and subsequent autonomy. The object relations model that is incorporated into the Transference-Focused Psychotherapy for Adolescents (TFP-A) approach (to be described in Chapter 2) offers the potential to utilize these self-other interaction patterns in clinically useful ways when appropriate to the individual's treatment. The various features just reviewed can contribute to young persons' developing hypersensitivity to others' reactions and deficits in awareness and appreciation of others' thoughts, and when the situation overwhelms their adaptive ability, they develop primitive defenses. These narrow and rigid coping skills can limit their capacity to adapt in a mature fashion.

# Maltreatment and Pathological Narcissism

From the point of view of psychological structure, narcissistic PD and BPD are closely related. However, there are still important gaps in our knowledge regarding the developmental precursors of grandiose narcissism and vulnerable narcissism (Campbell and Miller 2011; Dickinson and Pincus 2003). Some studies report positive relationships between maltreatment and both grandiose and vulnerable narcissism (Khoury et al. 2019; Lyons-Ruth et al. 2013), while others suggest that parental coldness or intrusive behaviors contribute to the development of vulnerable narcissism, but not grandiose narcissism (Crowe et al. 2016). In another study, negative parenting such as inconsistent discipline and lack of supervision was found to be linked to vulnerable narcissism in 16- to 17-year-olds, while grandiose narcissism was associated more with parental investment and positive reinforcement (Mechanic and Barry 2015). Consistent with this, overvaluation, and not lack of warmth and affection, was found to predict grandiose narcissism in children ages 7–12 (Brummelman et al. 2015). Furthermore, role reversal, or *parentification*, in which the child is forced to adopt parental emotional roles and responsibilities (Haxhe 2016), has also been linked to narcissism (Jones and Wells 1996).

## Attachment

Attachment styles are considered to be the outcome of multiple repeated affective interactions between mother and infant. In this way, attachment reflects the repeated balance of positive and negative interactions in which the mother either responded adequately to the infant's affective communication and distress and acted as a secure base, helping the infant reestablish self-regulation, or responded in an intrusive, hostile, helpless, passive, or other noncontingent way, contributing to an escalation of distress or leaving the child in an intolerable state of heightened stress. Furthermore, studies of mother-infant affective communication, such as those of Daniel Stern (1995) and others (Beebe 1986; Lyons-Ruth 1999), demonstrate how repeated patterns of dyadic affective communication form the foundation for later constellations of expectancies of how another is likely to respond to particular affects. Stern argued that these expectancies will have an impact on how the infant (and later the child and adult) expresses his or her affects in dyadic contexts. For example, the infant who repeatedly experiences his mother as becoming overly intrusive when he signals that he is distressed may come to express his distress with a mixture of frustration in anticipation of a mother who will try and engage him in another activity before he is regulated. His mother, and later his partner or significant others, seeing his look of frustration or anger when he feels distressed, may feel confused about whether he wants to be comforted, and may be hesitant to offer help for fear of being rejected.

Attachment organization has long-range predictive value and is especially relevant for understanding BPD and the development of emotional regulation, self and other representations, and accompanying interpersonal relations. For example, in a longitudinal study ranging from infancy to early adulthood, the relationship between attachment disorganization and BPD symptoms in early adulthood was explained (mediated) through the impact of attachment disorganization on self representation and the implications of this in turn for BPD symptoms (Carlson et al. 2009).

Developmental challenges during adolescence involving investment in a social network—reliance on friends and partners rather than on family and parent—may be positively or negatively influenced by early attachment styles and self and other representations that are activated. For example, secure attachment styles and trust will facilitate the transitions associated with separation from the family and individuation when adolescents increasingly rely on their own friends and social networks for support. Adolescence may also provide ample opportunities to reexamine and reorganize representations of self and other and to address identity issues, as adolescents are confronted by the difficulties that insecure and disorganized attachment styles may contribute to in their interpersonal relationships.

In the therapeutic relationship, this pattern translates into a transference[1] in which the adolescent is reluctant to express a range of emotions, negative as well as good feelings, about a positive event that might have happened. Within our object relations model, this attachment pattern with the therapist can and should be jointly examined. Such an intervention leads the adolescent to reexamine his or her self-other constructions and the defenses that maintained them, and to use more mature cognitive strategies for self-reflection so as to consider alternative constructions of the adolescent's self and of his or her reality.

## Case 2: Chris

Chris, an intelligent 16-year-old with a borderline personality organization, significant narcissistic features, and depressed mood said he viewed his therapist as merely being "a brick wall." He said this perspective allowed him

---

[1]Kernberg defines *transference* as the repetition in the here-and-now of a dominant conflict of the past. This conflict is played out in different styles of relating with others. The experiences of the past, good and bad, thus get activated in the here-and-now and affect how the individual perceives current situations and how he or she reacts to these situations.

to express his anger and not be concerned about what the therapist thought or felt and for him to not be curious about the therapist as a person. Chris was committed to therapy but expressed the concern that if the therapist became real (he would insist, "You're not a real person to me"), he would not be able to tolerate it and would have to stop therapy. It was as if he could not imagine that a "real" other could accept these aspects of his presentation and still want to be with him.

A principal focus in the treatment became Chris's inability to feel pleasure despite his wish to do so. When appropriate to the discussion of the moment, the intermittent examination of the role played by the "brick wall" imagery as a defense and its role in the transference and meaning for other relationships led him to recognize his concern about others being jealous of him (and helped him to realize that he was jealous of others and that he did not have to continue to see them in some devalued manner, e.g., as idiots). It also allowed him to recognize his concern that others would want to ruin the good things if he allowed those things to happen and be seen. In due course, he also started to think about his difficulty in receiving from or giving to others. (For example, gifting was a source of significant worry—receiving a gift meant a demand for reciprocity; giving would raise the concern that it might not be good enough.)

Of interest is that the "brick wall" concept could be returned to with some frequency over the course of months and utilized by Chris and his therapist to examine self-other constructions that contributed to enhancing his understanding and clarification of fears and expectations in relationships, while allowing him a degree of safety and distance.

# Multiple Pathways to BPD in Adolescence

As is evident from the preceding section, adolescents and young people who are diagnosed with BPD are not a unitary group. Adolescents who have quite different symptom profiles according to DSM criteria may meet criteria for the diagnosis of BPD, as is the case with adults. Research instruments also reflect the diversity among these young people. For example, the BPRC scale utilized by Belsky et al. (2012), derived from the Shedler-Westen Assessment Procedure–200 for Adolescents (SWAP-200-A) (Westen et al. 2003), reflects three fundamental features of adult BPD (affective instability/dysregulation, impulsivity/behavioral dysregulation, disturbed relatedness/interpersonal dysfunction). Specific items of the BPRC scale include "easily jealous"; "falls for new friends intensely"; "changes friends constantly"; "fears he/she will be rejected or abandoned"; "feels others are out to get him/her"; "acts overly seductive or sexy"; "emotions spiral out of control, has extremes of rage, despair, excitement"; "cannot think when upset, becomes irrational"; "unable to sooth or comfort self"; "lacks stable image of self, changes goals/values"; "expresses emotions in an exaggerated dramatic ways"; "irritable, touchy, or quick to fly off the handle"; "angry and hostile"; and "engages in self-harm behavior." It is not difficult to imagine that different adolescents with BPD can have different feature patterns and different developmental histories as well. Clinical experience also suggests the existence of qualitatively different groups of adolescents for whom the diagnosis of BPD is useful and appropriate.

Those adolescents who successfully navigate through the demands of adolescence, despite their ups and downs with parents and peers, demonstrate continuity of personality and convey the sense that they are building on their childhood selves rather than reinventing themselves. Even as they become more independent and develop views and values that are differentiated from those of their parents, they maintain their relationships with parents and family members. In addition, even when they develop views and values that differ and in some cases are in conflict with those of their parents, they maintain a certain capacity to see past these differences and appreciate positive aspects of the parents and are able to turn to their parents for help in times of need.

In contrast, the vast majority of adolescents who are diagnosed with BPD have childhood histories of long-standing and marked difficulties in affect and behavior regulation. One group whose symptoms frequently meet criteria for BPD during adolescence includes those who have shown relational disturbances involving inappropriate aggression directed toward others during childhood, such as ODD and CD.

Another group of adolescents with BPD may have a consistent pattern of inflexible and maladaptive reactions but do not display the problems of affect dysregulation and aggression associated with ODD or CD. These maladaptive qualities might be difficult to observe in situations that are structured, nonchallenging, or predictable. They are more likely to appear in periods of change and stress—for example, in the transition between middle school and high school; during activities that make greater interpersonal demands, such as making new friends and establishing a level of intimacy in a relationship; in situations involving challenges, competition, and the risk of failure and humiliation, such as taking tests, team sports, or performing publicly at school; or in situations that make new demands for autonomy, such as attending a sleepover, finding a job, and performing a job in the absence of supervision. Consistent maladaptive reactions to these activities and situations may be indicative of disturbances in characteristic defenses and coping mechanisms, and these underlying difficulties will become more and more evident at each developmental period so that there may be definite but less flamboyant evolution toward a PD when the individual is faced with the inevitable challenges of adolescence to separate, become more independent, and establish social and intimate relationships outside of the security of the family.

Adolescents who develop eating disorders or engage in self-harm frequently have such apparently unremarkable childhood histories. At most, they may have been somewhat sensitive, dependent, submissive, and obsessive as children. It is fair to conclude, though, that these adolescents, like those with ODD and CD, have long-standing difficulties that are entrenched in their personalities but that become increasingly evident in the context of demands to become autonomous and take on increasing responsibilities and make decisions, while separating from parents and developing new intimate relationships.

There is another small group of adolescents without obvious childhood psychological problems or personality difficulties who may display an identity crisis that is difficult to distinguish from BPD in adolescence. These young people have difficulty preserving a sense of continuity and coherence when their capacities for adaptation are overwhelmed by the challenges that often accompany adolescence. The longitudinal trajectory study of self-esteem by Birkeland et al. (2012) included some individuals that may be representative of this group of adolescents. The self-esteem of a group representing approximately 7% of adolescents in the study was described by a U-shaped trajectory in which initially good self-esteem decreased markedly between ages 14 and 18 years and reached its lowest level in late adolescence, before improving during the next 5 years. The adolescents in this group may have had preexisting fragilities that compromised their capacity to adapt to change and their difficulties during adolescence, despite the apparently improved self-esteem, may have led to some kind of scarring, because their global self-esteem at age 30 was significantly lower than that of individuals with consistently high self-esteem during adolescence. They also presented with significantly higher levels of depression. This would suggest that adolescents who experience identity crisis or sharp decreases in self-esteem may also warrant intervention and potentially derive significant long-term benefits from therapy. The therapeutic intervention needs to be sensitive to the presence of a PD and not just view the difficulties as manifestations of a depressive disorder.

Another group comprises those who are victims of sexual abuse. Sexual abuse just before or at the beginning of adolescence may be particularly destabilizing. It can be the final blow for girls who had shown resilient personality characteristics and who were able to continue to function well at school and invest in friendships despite parental neglect, substance abuse, psychological problems, and immaturity. Although many PTSD symptoms can be expected to resolve in due course, sexual abuse may interfere with the capacity of adolescent girls to form intimate relationships and to develop trust in partners.

Adolescents who engage in increased risk taking, especially when drugs, alcohol, and sex are involved, may also be at higher risk of presenting with identity crisis and lowered self-esteem when they develop addictions, experience trauma, or become overwhelmed when their behaviors take them down paths for which they are unprepared.

Another group that may be particularly at risk are those adolescents who are confronted with the task of assuming a sexual identity that is not culturally desirable and involves the possibility of being alienated from peers and family.

Breakdown and identity diffusion that presents like BPD can be seen in hypersensitive adolescents when there is parental separation, especially when the separation is accompanied by conflict and geographical moves to distant cities that make parents less available. These circumstances can also be associated with a loss of friends, and the adolescent is challenged to integrate into a new social circle and adapt to a new academic environment. This may be associated with the onset of suicidal/self-harming behavior.

Parental mental illness and chaotic family environments, in which parents respond with inappropriate physical aggression to adolescent self-assertion and bids for separation, can also lead to breakdowns that result in identity diffusion in sensitive or vulnerable adolescents.

# Adolescence as a Critical Period for Development of Personality Disorders

BPD symptoms typically appear in adolescence and peak from ages 14 to 17 years and then gradually decline (Arens et al. 2013; Bornovalova et al. 2009; Chanen and Kaess 2012). Even when symptoms like impulsivity tend to decline, underlying negative affect and feelings of emptiness are more likely to persist (Meares et al. 2011). Also, according to the Children in the Community (CIC) Study (Cohen et al. 2005), high symptom levels of any personality disorder in adolescence have negative repercussions on functioning over the subsequent 10–20 years, and these repercussions are often more serious or pervasive than those associated with Axis I disorders. The same study also found that some youth manifest an increase in PD symptoms from mid-adolescence to early adulthood and that symptoms of BPD are the strongest predictors of later PD. Data from the CIC Study were used to investigate the relationship between early BPD symptoms and subsequent psychosocial functioning. They demonstrated an association of early BPD symptoms with less productive adult role functioning, lower educational attainment and occupational status in middle adulthood, an adverse effect on relationship quality, and lower adult life satisfaction (Winograd et al. 2008). Elevated BPD symptoms in adolescence have been shown to be an independent risk factor for substance use disorders during early adulthood (Cohen et al. 2007).

There are many reasons why BPD symptoms may first become apparent in adolescence. Most apparent is that this pattern is attributable to developmental changes in brain structures, with the decline in BPD symptoms associated with maturation of control mechanisms (Powers and Casey 2015). Also physical, cognitive, and social changes may contribute to its onset during that period.

# Neurobiological Changes in Adolescence

Transformations occur across adolescence and extend into early adulthood. They include brain changes in the frontal lobe regions that contribute to the marked growth in higher-order abstract reasoning, problem solving, decision making, and mentalization. Yet, despite the rapid development of these abilities, adolescents seem more emotionally reactive and vulnerable to making bad decisions, and go against their better judgment and engage in risky behaviors, especially when under the influence of emotions and peers. Casey and Jones (2010) have proposed an "imbalance model" to describe adolescent brain development, whereby the limbic system is functionally mature at a time when the prefrontal systems are still developing, leaving the adolescent more susceptible to the influence of the reward-sensitive limbic system. Adults too, as described by a dual processing model, use reflexive or automatic, intuitive, affect-driven heuristic processes, mediated by subcortical systems, although they are capable of more reflective, controlled rational processes subserved by the prefrontal cortex (PFC) (Evans et al. 2002; Galvan 2012; Reyna 2004; Reyna and Farley 2006; Romer et al. 2017). In the dual systems model, decisions result from an interaction between more thoughtful processes and more experienced-based, affective, heuristic, and motivational processes (Damasio 1994a, 1994b; Epstein 1994; Evans 2008; Lerner and Keltner 2000; M.D. Lieberman 2000; Loewenstein et al. 2001; Schneider and Caffray 2012, Stanovich and West 2000). BPD pathology in adults and adolescents, including dysregulated negative affect, impulsive and aggressive behavior, and interpersonal difficulties, can be seen as derived from deficits in these reflective and executive control processes, coupled with a biased reflexive process in which there is an automatic hypersensitivity to negative social cues (Koenigsberg et al. 2009), an expectation of untrustworthiness (King-Casas et al. 2008), and increased negative affect (Sadikaj et al. 2010).

Casey (2015) provides a more detailed developmental analysis of the changing interrelationship during adolescence among the PFC, ventral striatum, and the amygdala that offers a framework for understanding several of the behavioral features that seem to characterize adolescents. The PFC, as a mediator of reasoning and behavioral regulation processes, can suppress output for both the ventral striatum and amygdala. As the functioning of these areas becomes more coordinated over time, there is a greater integration of cognitive and emotional processes, which results in increased motivated and goal-oriented actions. However, the development of the PFC extends through adolescence, whereas the ventral striatum and amygdala reach more mature functioning at an earlier time; therefore, behaviors that require greater self-control (e.g., focusing attention on relevant information and withdrawing attention from irrelevant but possibly interesting information) suffer, compared with later adolescence and early adulthood. As an illustration of a function that would have clinical importance, the ventral striatum is more responsive to larger rewards than to smaller ones in mid-adolescence when compared with childhood and adulthood, and as a result 15-year-olds are more likely than adults to make risky gambles for immediate reward feedback (Casey 2015). In general, adolescents are more impulsive responders to positive cues than are children or adults.

The presence of peers is associated with even riskier decision making (Steinberg 2008). It is not that adolescents lack the knowledge to make the wiser choice; rather, adolescents appear to be especially sensitive to incentives (e.g., money, peer acceptance) and contexts, such as the presence of peers, that seem to heighten motivational states. Therefore, the adolescent will be less likely to suppress inappropriate actions and desires when the context includes salient cues because their capacity for response regulation is still incompletely developed. Casey (2015) also noted that drug use may interact with the dopamine system and heighten responsivity in the ventral striatum, thereby strengthening the reward properties of the drug during a phase when the PFC and its associated control mechanisms are still immature.

Casey (2015) indicated that the changes she described in adolescence are found across species, and so it may be that the movement from dependence to autonomy is greatly aided by the increase in novelty seeking and peer interactions found among adolescents. The increased value of incentives and the wish to obtain more resources and new sexual experiences may enhance the movement out of the home and support the separation-individuation process. She noted that adolescence may be thought of as "a period of thrills and fears," but many of our patients have not found the balance to master the fear by using judgment in a manner that would also promote safe exploration and autonomy. Of clinical interest, during this period of neurological imbalance, adolescents show diminished fear extinction, which suggests that exposure procedures might be less effective, and, as Casey (2015) pointed out, there is some evidence for reduced treatment efficacy of cognitive-behavioral therapy in adolescence compared with children and adults. One possible mechanism in TFP-A interventions that could contribute to their effectiveness is support of ego functioning, providing a form of scaffolding that helps the adolescent compensate for cognitive immaturities.

# Puberty

Puberty takes several years from onset to completion, and hormonal changes precede the observable physical changes. The process typically begins earlier in girls than in boys. The physical changes include the development of secondary sexual characteristics (e.g., pubic hair growth; breast and penile development) and a growth spurt; changes in body shape, size, and composition; and menarche/spermarche. These observable changes signal that the developing young person is entering a new phase in life, and this transition brings with it new expectations and reactions from parents, siblings, and peers, aside from reactions of the young person whenever he or she looks in a mirror. What is often clinically relevant is the degree of synchrony between the adolescent's experience of physical and personal maturity and the granting of social maturity and autonomy by the family and society (Rudolph 2014).

Pubertal status can be associated with features of psychopathology such as an increase in anxiety, depression, antisocial behavior, and problematic substance use during the pubertal transition (Rudolph 2014). There is also

a heightened reactivity to emotions and information with emotional conno-
tations during this period, and cognitive control is more readily undermined by salient emotional information and incentives (Silk et al. 2009).
Early maturation may serve to exacerbate already existing individual differences in vulnerability to psychopathology, and of value to the clinician's understanding is that assessment in early adolescence (11–13 years) can be a
better predictor of adult functioning than assessment of similar behaviors
made in younger children or in middle adolescence (Livson and Peskin 1967).
Perhaps individual differences become magnified across periods of change,
such as during pubertal transition, as these periods of biological transformation also evoke demands for social and intrapsychic change, and the greater
inter-individual variability during such periods of change allows for greater
predictive utility.

Many studies have focused on the timing of pubertal changes—are they
early or late occurring, and does the timing have a differential effect on boys
and girls? It appears that there are advantages and disadvantages to early
and late maturing for boys and girls. Although it is usually thought that early
maturation is advantageous for boys, conferring heightened social status
and respect, it is also the case that early-maturing boys may feel out of sync
with their age and grade mates and are thus more likely to enter into social
relations with older boys who are more likely to engage in risky and norm-
breaking behavior at a time when the early maturers are not emotionally or
cognitively prepared to handle it. For early-maturing girls, risky, pseudo-
mature sexual behavior may also occur. They, and later-maturing boys, may
be more likely to experience internalizing problems and depressive symptoms. For girls, high-for-age hormonal levels are associated with depressive
features, including sadness.

# Sexuality, Identity, and Early Experience

Changes in sexuality and aggression associated with puberty demand integration into personal identity and necessitate learning how to express these
drives in interpersonal and intimate contexts. Sexual attraction and desire
for someone pulls and pushes adolescents to develop intimate experiences
and relationships outside of the family, forcing them to face an ensuing
sense of elation combined with loss. The change from being physically
childlike to accepting a new physical self that is at once experiencing new
sensations and functional capacities and also capable of feeling and eliciting

sexual desire may be challenging for any adolescent to integrate at the level of identity. The continuous body changes will, alternatively and in waves, either confuse or confirm the adolescent's identity feelings. At the same time the relationship with family and peers may become sexualized. Sexual desire for another on the one hand and being desired on the other hand propel adolescents into exploring new experiences involving physical and emotional intimacy with others outside the family. In an entirely novel setting they have to negotiate the experience of being close to someone else when there are the threats of rejection as well as regression and fusion. Sexual experiences also challenge the adolescent to develop control of aggression and impulsivity; consider the needs, desires, and feelings of another in an intimate physical context; and discover new ways of communication to manage the vulnerability of each of the adolescent partners. Masturbatory activity continues to offer an outlet for self-soothing and also provides a means for learning and practicing the expression and control of sexual action.

Preadolescent experiences impact the young person's integration of sexual and aggressive demands into a developing sense of self. For adolescents who have experienced sexual abuse or sexualization, or for adolescents who have conflicts or confusion regarding their sexual identity, the unavoidable confrontation with sexuality during adolescence may strain and threaten the cohesion and continuity of their sense of self.

For adolescents with extremely difficult and painful attachment histories whose early experiences of intimacy have been marked by fear, hostility, frustration, intrusiveness, rejection, abandonment, and helplessness, sexual intimacy is likely to re-evoke these deep anxieties with associated fears around dependency, regressive fusion, aggression, shame, and abandonment. So, as they experience a novel, heretofore unique, extrafamilial relationship, the desire for closeness and their first sexual experiences may, in vulnerable adolescents, trigger deep anxieties and crises that challenge their fragile sense of self and bring to the forefront weaknesses in the self that may not have been so evident during childhood.

Adolescents with histories of sexual abuse may also feel particularly vulnerable. The traumatic experiences and feelings related to the abuse intrude into their first sexual relationship, and this makes it more complex and challenging for them to integrate this experience into their identities. In addition, vulnerable adolescents with personality pathology may fail to assert and protect themselves sufficiently and are less likely to anticipate and avoid potentially dangerous interpersonal situations; they also may consume drugs and alcohol so that they are more likely to have nonconsensual and traumatic sexual experiences in adolescence that may destabilize them further.

Adolescents who have been sexualized prematurely, whether through sexualized mother-infant or toddler contact or through lack of parental boundaries or controls around witnessing sexual intercourse, may also be particularly vulnerable and may require additional help to understand these experiences and their consequences in order to better integrate into their identity their engagement in sexual behavior and promiscuity.

The issues of sexual orientation and gender identity can provoke anxiety and be a major source of deep conflict in adolescence while straining the capacity to integrate aspects of the self that may be experienced as alien and dangerous, and may lead to breakdown and serious suicide attempts. While adolescence is a period when the boundaries between friendship and sexual attraction may blur, confronting the adolescent with their potential for bisexual or same-gender sexual attraction, for the vast majority of adolescents this is a passing phase that does not result in undue anxiety. However, for adolescents who are confronted by the homosexual nature of their attractions, it is frequently challenging to integrate this awareness into their identities. This is further complicated when it is their first sexual experience, potentially testing their personality's cohesion and capacity for flexibility. It also tests their sense of independence, to see if they will experience and then can survive parental, familial, peer, and societal rejection or disappointment. For adolescents without a strong sense of self, the anxieties and conflicts stirred up by discovering a sexual orientation not accepted by their family or community could lead to personality crisis.

## Cognitive Changes

It is also interesting to consider the possible contribution of the development of abstract thinking during adolescence, which of course is also subject to neurodevelopmental and genetic contributions. Therefore, we might expect that for those who show a continuance of BPD symptoms over the adolescence period—namely, those for whom it is not a stage-specific phenomenon (cf. Moffitt 1993a, 1993b)—more is involved than the contribution of advanced abstract thinking, and the crisis is not normative. In the normative condition, it is less likely that PD features such as true splitting would be seen.

# Summary

BPD, as well as narcissistic, antisocial, and avoidant PDs, can be diagnosed in adolescence. A reluctance to diagnose BPD in young people may increases the risk of more severe outcomes because it reduces access to psychotherapy. Psychotherapy that addresses personality disturbance is essential to help adolescents resume engagement with developmental challenges in a way that can facilitate personality development. There are likely multiple pathways to BPD, consistent with the concept of equifinality. In addition, there may be several "subtypes" of adolescent BPD as a function of varied developmental histories, and there may be many experiences before and during adolescence that can compromise the process of identity formation.

In a TFP-A model, difficulties at the level of identity formation constitute a core feature of BPD. Contributions to the development of BPD come from genetic, temperamental, and experiential forces in interaction with one another. So, although these pathways are somewhat nonspecific, perhaps the common factor is that they impact parent-child interactions and the nature of the attachment relationship and other ensuing relationships. This, in turn, impacts the development of the growing child's sense of self, which together with the developmental demands of adolescence, shapes identity formation, the bedrock of personality and PDs.

In the next chapter, we present a contemporary psychodynamic conceptualization of PDs in adolescence as well as structural changes and developmental challenges that are hypothesized to be disrupted and sidetracked because of the core problem of PDs, which is identity diffusion.

# CHAPTER 2

# Psychodynamic Conceptualization of Personality, Development, and Personality Disorders at Adolescence

**ADOLESCENCE** is a phase of major structural changes and indicative of the advancing instinctual, physical, neurological, mental, and intellectual maturation processes. At a psychodynamic level, it is a period between a saddening farewell to childhood—that is, to the old self and the objects of the past—and a gradual, anxious eagerness to pass over many barriers to the unknown territory of adulthood. Beginning with their childhood love objects, adolescents must not only free themselves from persons who were all-important during childhood, but renounce their former pleasures and get on to new challenges more rapidly than at any former developmental stage. Constructing a new image of themselves due to the psychophysiological sexual development associated with the rapid and visible body changes and liberated sexual and hostile impulses, adolescents must prepare to leave home sooner or later and become independent and autonomous; to become skilled at adult sexuality, love, and responsibility; to form new personal, intimate, and social relations of different types; to develop new interests and sublimations; and, last but not least, to assimilate new values, standards, ethics, and ideals that will offer them directions for the future and help in making crucial decisions such as their career choice, which will determine their work and future financial and social situation, and choice of a love object. Since this period involves processes of renunciation and integration of new and sometimes opposite desires and ideals, it is not surprising that for a briefer or longer period of time these processes of transformation will cause marked fluctuations in adolescents' general functioning and in their behavior, and not only disturb their relations to their parents and their object relations in general but transform their personality and identity.

These major changes have four important implications for the treatment of adolescents. First, even though the majority of adolescents are adaptable and overcome these developmental stressors without significant difficulties and resume a normal course of development, many others are less flexible or are confronted with traumatic experiences at this specific phase of development. Thus, the therapist may find it difficult to distinguish normality from abnormality in this confusion of emotional manifestations and symptomatology associated with this phase. Anna Freud (1958) has compared the struggle of the adolescent to the "mourning process," in which the individual shows sudden mood swings or passes through sometimes violent and peculiar affective crises that may involve severe guilt conflicts, and distressing feelings of shame and self-consciousness to the point of hypochondriacal body preoccupations or paranoid fears. One week the adolescent may be in a state of depressing sadness and despair. The next week he may encounter a period of intense concentration and introspection, sharing his enthusiasm and burning interest in a new activity or his studies. But these behaviors may again be followed by a period of secret, risky behaviors or overwhelming doubts.

Also, as Winnicott (1962/1965; Winnicott et al. 1984) noted, adolescence alters the shape of psychiatric illness. Indeed, some adolescents who have normal functioning may show antisocial tendencies or like to be grouped together with troubled individuals or offer help to the most depressed on the fringe of the group to give reality to their own potential symptomatology. Alternatively, it is not rare to see adolescents with borderline personality disorder (BPD) taking on responsibilities far beyond what is expected for their age, as with the adolescent who takes charge of her siblings in an alcoholic family. On the whole, the boys and girls making up the first group will come through adolescence without suicide, violence, theft, or prostitution. In the second group, the adolescent girl who takes charge of her siblings may express fragile resilience that will protect her from developing a pathology, while the adolescent boy's "potential health" from a brief hospitalization may not stand for health itself and may need proper long-term treatment. Guidelines to distinguish normal from abnormal development are therefore taken into consideration in Transference-Focused Psychotherapy for Adolescents (TFP-A).

Second, as inferred from the above, adolescence is also a stage of tremendous instinctual-narcissistic striving that opposes reaching out for help and therapeutic support. This stage coincides with the period during which the "ideal ego," seen as the nostalgic survival of the lost infantile narcissism and its felt omnipotence, is transformed into the "ego ideal," seen as a dynamic and realistic formation that sustains ambitions toward progress as well as acceptance of imperfections and limited power and capacities. This, in our view, explains different forms of resistances to treatment, especially for pre-adolescents and young adolescents who oscillate between those two states accompanied either by self-importance, bragging, arrogance, and mutism or by self-depreciation, self-effacement, shame, or guilt. Technical modifications in TFP-A (introduced later in this manual) are therefore made to take into consideration this highly sensitive, narcissistic attitude toward the therapist and the treatment.

Third, some adolescents enter adolescence already weakened and vulnerable or unambiguously distressed by an established personality disorder (PD). The presence of PDs is hypothesized to derail or preclude the generally expectable developmental pathways of adolescence and more specifically the personality organization and identity integration. Our experience has led us to notice that as much as PDs affect the development of the adolescent, it is nonetheless the case that not all developmental structures are affected, not at the same level, and that some structures persist that develop quasi-normally, sometimes embryonically or hidden by the more primitive and underdeveloped ones in the foreground. It is our belief that there exists an interaction between maturational and pathological processes. It is also our belief that to be effective in treating PDs at adolescence, a therapist must keep in mind a model of understanding the PD's pathology and the related aims of a treatment and a model of normal development with its corresponding structural changes and challenges that the adolescent will inevitably have to face, successfully or not. This will permit the therapist to be sensitive to what is typical and what is atypical in the adolescent's behaviors and relationships as well as to "preview" and to "focus on" imminent maturational trends, structural changes in the personality organization, and developmental challenge ahead. TFP-A is a psychodynamic treatment of PDs grounded into a developmental perspective.

Fourth, and finally, as seen in the previous chapter, the reflective and executive control processes, located in the prefrontal zone of the brain, mature and establish themselves at a slower pace than does the one-sided reflexive process of the limbic area. This difference in maturation has psychodynamic implications in the sense that the typically developing adolescent's mentalization capacities are not fully accessible before mid-adolescence, and for adolescents with PDs, the PD is even more debilitating and incapacitating because of their automatic hypersensitivity to negative social cues, expectation of untrustworthiness, and intense negative affects. For some of them, the interpretative process of TFP-A may give them enough perspective to regulate their affects and impulses, but for others, more disturbed and afflicted, some psychoeducation techniques may be necessary to help them to pay attention, to gain perspective, and to mentalize self and other's experiences. The use of metaphor can also facilitate mentalization capacities because the appropriate image or metaphor can mirror or evoke feelings in the patient in a way that facilitates empathic attunement. If feelings can then be objectified, their power to distress or overwhelm is mitigated. Indeed, Kernberg (2015) mentioned that significant learning occurs under conditions of activation of "low affective states," as opposed to "peak affect state" (i.e., when direct perception and cognitive elaboration of the perceived environment permit cognitive learning relatively uninfluenced by the expression of organismic needs reflected in affect activation). Metaphor objectifies and bypasses the activation of peak affect traces.

We have to remember also that reflective functioning and formal operational reasoning (Piaget 1972), associated with the ability for abstract reasoning or with imagined realities that are different from the current one, are two different constructs, located in two different areas of the brain, and even though they may interact, the successful functioning of the former is necessary for the full use of the latter in situations of peak negative affects and perceived malevolent intentions. This is why even brilliant adolescents may look extremely concrete and unintelligent in their analysis of a highly affective situation. Or, some adolescents feel that they have all the time in the world or that there is not enough time to do what they need to do. They may languish and remain inactive, as they see some of their peers moving on in their development toward adulthood, because they may experience a sense of time or work diffusion due to an incapacity for self-reflection—and not necessarily because they are lacking the capacity to project themselves into the future or to analyze opportunities.

We will now present the components of personality that undergo major reorganization at adolescence and describe the structural changes as well as challenges expected to happen at adolescence that are derived from normal maturational processes. This will constitute the basis of a developmental model to be used by the therapist as a template to compare, predict, and foresee manifested behaviors and level of functioning. It will also serve to measure structural change. We will then present a contemporary psychody-

---

**TABLE 2–1.**  **Features of personality organization from the Inventory of Personality Organization–Adolescent Version (IPO-A)**

---

Sense of Self or Other (Identity): Confusion ↔ Diffusion

Quality of Object Relations: Good, Preserved ↔ Poor, unstable

Maturity of Defenses: Mature ↔ Primitive

Reality Testing: Preserved ↔ Questionable (psychotic-like)

Moral Functioning: Rebellious, Individualized ↔ Rigid, persecutory, Self-righteousness

Aggressivity: In the service of autonomy ↔ In the service of destruction or regression

Sexuality: In the service of embodied-self, intimacy and love ↔ Inhibition, Promiscuity

*Self-Esteem: Healthy narcissism ↔ Vulnerable or Grandiose Narcissism

*Separation: Autonomy, Individuation ↔ Failure to launch, Flight into adulthood

---

*New edition of the IPO-A (in revision).

namic object relations theory to explain PDs and introduce the construct of identity diffusion that is hypothesized to be the core feature of PD manifestations. This will constitute the basis of a pathological model to be used by the therapist to identify the focus of his or her interventions.

# Structural Changes at Adolescence and Developmental Challenges

The period of adolescence is relatively uneventful for the vast majority of adolescents. They follow a normal development in which there is a consolidation and strengthening of identity. Abnormal development can occur when there is a derailing in some or all of the key dimensions of personality organization. These dimensions include a sense of self and other, quality of object representation, defenses (from primitive to mature), reality testing, moral functioning, aggressivity, sexuality, narcissism, and separation (Table 2–1). Our research findings suggests that three groups can be differentiated using these domains—namely, a normal developing group with none or few problems in any of these domains, a second group who have difficulties in self and other representations who we consider to present with identity crisis, and a third group who have difficulties in multiple domains that are indicative of personality disorder (Biberdzic et al. 2018).

During the assessment process, while implementing therapeutic interventions, and when determining the status of the psychotherapy progress, including termination decisions, the therapist working with adolescents continually faces the question of distinguishing between the vicissitudes of normal adolescence and manifestations of psychopathology of that age period. The understanding of structural changes and developmental challenges that happen at adolescence constitutes a template to compare, predict, and foresee expected behaviors and level of functioning and to distinguish normal from abnormal development.

# Contemporary Object Relations Theory

The TFP-A model of PDs considers the adolescent's observable behaviors and subjective disturbances to reflect pathological features of underlying psychological structures. A *psychological structure* is a stable and enduring pattern of mental functions that organizes the individual's behavior, perceptions, and subjective experience. A fundamental characteristic of the psychological organization of adolescents with severe personality disorders is the lack of an integrated conceptualization of self and of significant others, which is called the syndrome of *identity diffusion*. The individual's level of personality organization is seen as reflecting the degree of integration of these personality structures.

Object relations theory emphasizes that the drives described by Sigmund Freud—libido and aggression—are always experienced in relation to a specific object of the drive, or "other." Internal object relations are constructs that represent the building blocks of the individuals's internal world, the psychological structure that serves as the organizer of motivation and behavior. These basic building blocks of psychic structure are units made up of a representation of the self, an affect related to or representing a drive, and a representation of the other (the object of the drive). These units of self, other, and the affect linking them are referred to as *object relations dyads* (Figure 2–1). It is important to note that the "self" and the "object" in the dyad are not accurate, actual internal representations of the entirety of the self or the other, but rather representations of the self and other as they were experienced in specific moments in time in the course of early development in pri-

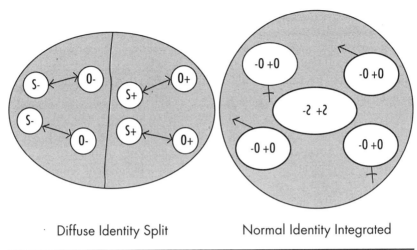

Diffuse Identity Split            Normal Identity Integrated

**FIGURE 2–1.   Representation of dyadic units of internalized object relations.**

mary attachment relationships, that may have been defensively distorted because of the impact of wishes, fears, or anxieties in the course of intrapsychic development.

The adult with a normal personality organization has developed an integrated concept of self and of significant others that is captured in the concept of identity. This concept includes both a coherent internal sense of self and a pattern of behavior that reflects self coherence. Such coherence of self is basic to self-esteem, enjoyment, and the capacity to derive pleasure from relationships with others and from commitment to work, school, or other responsibilities. A coherent and integrated sense of self contributes to the realization of one's capabilities, desires, and long-range goals. Likewise, a coherent and integrated conception of others contributes to a realistic evaluation of others, utilizing empathy and social tact. An integrated sense of self and significant others permits the development of intimacy and stability in love relationships and the harmonious integration of tenderness and eroticism in such relationships.

A basic assumption of contemporary object relations theory is that all internalizations of relationships with significant others, from the beginning of life on, have different characteristics under the conditions of peak affect interactions and low affect interactions. Under conditions of peak affect activation—be they of an extremely positive, pleasurable mode or an extremely negative, painful mode—specific internalizations take place framed by the dyadic nature of the interaction between the baby and the caretaking person, resulting in specific positive and negative affective memory structures with powerful motivational implications. These early positive and negative affective memories are segregated in the mind, building up separately into two split-off segments, dissociated from each other in a way that maintains a domain reflecting an ideal self-other relation that is separate and protected from the frightening experiences of negative aggressive and punitive affect states. These negative affect states tend to be projected and seen as originating outside the self, creating the fear of "bad" external objects, whereas the totally positive affect states evolve into the memory of moments of a relationship with "ideal" objects and the wish for a permanent reunion with and realization of this state. In the course of early development, this results in two major, mutually split domains of early psychic experience in all individuals. The idealized one reflects a sense of purely positive representations of self and other, and the negative one reflects persecutory or paranoid representations of the other and a threatened representation of the self. This early split protects the wished-for idealized representations of self and other from "contamination" and potential destruction by bad ones until a higher degree of tolerance of pain and a more realistic assessment of external reality under painful conditions evolve in the course of normal development.

Eventually, the development of greater cognitive sophistication and the learning of realistic aspects of self and others interacting under circumstances of low affect activation foster in the young child the integration of these two peak affect–determined segments into more realistic and complex, rich and nuanced representations of self and others. Most individuals develop psychologically with a predominance of positive idealized experiences, and this allows for tolerating awareness of the negative charged internal representations of self and other, leading to the ability to integrate into the broader sense of self. This integration neutralizes their impact to a large degree and results in a marked diminishing of the paranoid fears and anxieties that resulted from the projection of these internal images of self and other. In simple terms, under healthy developmental conditions in which the good aspects predominate, there occurs an integration and neutralization of the paranoid element, and the child comes to recognize that he or she has both "good' and "bad" aspects, and so does mother and significant others, resulting in an integrated view of self and others. This advancement, which characterizes the separation-individuation process, referred to by Kleinian authors (Klein 1940; Segal 1964) as the shift from the paranoid-schizoid to the depressive position and by ego psychological authors as the shift into object constancy, is theorized to take place as a gradual integration over the first 3 years of life (Mahler 1972a, 1972b).

# Separation-Individuation Process

The separation-individuation process that began in the earliest years, resulting in object constancy, leads to the establishment of the sense "that I am." Adolescence can be seen as requiring a second individuation phase (Blos 1962) and the establishment of "what I am/what I might be." The adolescent, aided by the maturational advances derived from the physiological and neurological changes of the period, begins to move "out of the nest," ideally supported by parental recognition and acceptance of their child's changes as well as acceptance of societal expectations about the meaning of these changes and the required transition toward greater autonomy. The progressive separation from parents and family and the deeper investment in peers, romantic interests, and thoughts about work, career, and independent functioning contribute to and are aided by two primary tasks of adolescence: 1) the development of individual identity and 2) the capacity for intimacy.

A core sense of self that will be recognized as meaningful by others takes form as the adolescent begins to rework attachments and identifications with parents, friends, teachers, and significant others, including identifications with social class, ethnic and religious groups, and gender, while also integrating alterations in body image, sexuality, and new responsibilities. So, too, adolescents must renounce former pleasures and pursuits, and as they prepare to separate from home during adolescence as they approach adulthood, they must learn to reach out for increasingly mature sexuality, love, and responsibility; for personal and social relations of a new and different type; for new interests and sublimations; and for new values, standards, and goals. This process necessitates a reorientation that leads to structural and energic transformations, redistributions of emotional investment, and psychic reorganization, and these substantial transformations contribute to the shifting mood and emotional turmoil often shown by adolescents. These developmental accomplishments allow the adolescent to develop and sustain an intimate relationship that balances self-gratification with the desire and ability to satisfy another's needs. At a sexual level, an intimate relation is characterized by the ability to combine tenderness, sexuality, and romance, as well as aggression and competition. These developmental accomplishments require successfully moving away from parents along with developing a more mature, sustainable connection with them. Doing so helps the adolescent become able to maintain attachments to others without fear of rejection.

The adolescent with BPD, showing the impact of the split between the good and bad object-world, struggles to maintain a strong attachment to another, but often the fear of being rejected or engulfed jeopardizes the relation, preventing true closeness, trust, and mutual support, and instead results in threats to end the relationship and rapid or frequent transitions in relationships.

# Case 1: Jack

Jack, a 17-year-old, very intelligent high school senior, struggled throughout his academic career to complete schoolwork at a level commensurate with his ability. Whenever he faced a developmental demand (e.g., completing schoolwork, developing friendships, going off to summer camp, applying to colleges), he would blame his parents for constraining him and "ruining" his life, and he would often point to what he thought were his mother's inadequacies and blame her for preventing him from being successful. In effect he would project blame and failure onto his parents, create adolescent versions of tantrums, but not allow himself the freedom to master these demands and truly separate. At the same time, this defensive style contributed to an inability to allow for intimacy and experience pleasure, characterized by him as "emptiness," as is often reported by individuals with BPD. Under the guise of wishing to be free of controlling parents, he exerted a forceful omnipotent control that prevented true separation, individuation, and autonomous mastery of age-expected goals and prevented closeness with others, thereby thwarting the gratification of normal dependency needs and preventing him from asking for or receiving help from others, be it family, teachers, or peers. He argued that he wanted to be left alone but effectively manipulated his anxious parents' vigilance and counter-control. Thus, the parents became the anxious ones, were enraged, and were threatening to abandon him, while the young man clamored for independence yet prevented its occurrence. This stance maintained a narcissistic self that aspired to greatness but avoided confronting demands of life because "why bother if you can't be number one [and you cannot be number one if your parents prevent that]."

An objective of TFP-A is to foster the integration of developmentally earlier and more recent affective or motivational systems involving aggression, sexuality, dependency, autonomy, and morality, a goal often approached by examining object relations as reflected in extratransferential and transferential content. For example, as in the clinical example above, the adolescent with an unintegrated identity may reject all of the therapist's comments, leaving the adolescent as the powerful, right one and the therapist as the bad, inadequate one. This allows the young patient to devalue and not accept what the therapist may have to offer him; to use his sessions, which were reliably attended, "to vent"; and to prevent a level of intimacy and expression of warmth from emerging or, if it does, from showing. This reversal of the dyad lets the adolescent feel powerful and safe for the moment, but this use of the defense of omnipotent control, a manifestation of splitting, also prevents the adolescent from moving forward in the relationship with the therapist, preventing an integrated view of the therapist as someone who may make mistakes but also can be correct and as someone who offers nurturance and acceptance of the bad aspects of the self. This adolescent, while professing independence, is left feeling deprived and empty and envious of others who can ask, receive, and experience help and pleasure. Within this object relations model, it can be seen how the degree of identity integration promotes accurate self-reflection, comfort with interpersonal and sexual intimacy, less impairment in school/work performance, and positive self-esteem and why TFP-A offers a treatment model based on an integration of these elements in order to promote a more positive and mature sense of self and others. The therapist's effort in this process is aided by an understanding of identity formation.

# Identity

The utility of the construct of identity is broadly recognized and provides a central idea for understanding a wide range of human functioning (Schwartz et al. 2011). Kernberg's conceptualization of ego identity focuses on the "inner structural foundation of identity," and this feature is the "precondition for the many aspects of identity conceptualized by others" (Jørgensen 2010, p. 346). Empirical support for such a sweeping view is provided, for example, by an examination of the relationship among PD criteria that identified a general factor consisting primarily of BPD items, with identity disturbance being the core feature of this general factor (Sharp et al. 2015). The centrality of identity is also consistent with emerging models proposed in Section III of DSM-5 (American Psychiatric Association 2013) in which disturbances in self, which includes identity and self-direction, and disturbances in interpersonal functioning, which includes empathy and intimacy, are considered to be underlying features of all personality pathology. The emphasis on identity as the basic, underlying substrate of PDs is highly compatible with the assessment and treatment of adolescents, for whom identity formation may be the core developmental task (Erikson 1950).

Akhtar and Samuel (1996) have described the components of identity as including a realistic body image; an awareness of a core gender identity (male or female); gender roles (femininity or masculinity); sexual orientation (heterosexual or homosexual); a subjective self-sameness across situations; smooth transitions between various self representations emerging under diverse social circumstances; temporal continuity; a true capacity to recognize the positive and negative traits in one's self and in others that conveys a sense of authenticity; ethnic identity constituted of cultural values, verbal and nonverbal modes of expression, and patterns of interpersonal behaviors; and finally, a conscience that reflects the capacity to respond to rewards and punishments, to experience remorse and guilt, and to work toward ideals.

An integrated identity also involves a realistic view of significant others that tolerates the complex integration of positive and negative features of their personality, and the capacity to maintain such a view even under conditions of temporary conflict or mood that inflict negative affective interactions with them. For example, in the young man described earlier (see Case 3), over time he could state that his parents were good, caring people and that in many ways he was like them, but at other moments of peak affect, he would get angry and controlling and state that their involvement "in his life" felt "poisonous." This split representation felt to him to be in support of autonomy, but it actually prevented intimacy and resulted from his inflexibility. It is our opinion that school-age children have already attained a good level of integration of these components. Indeed, identity formation is a lifelong process that, as already noted, has its roots in children's earliest interactions with their environment. Children's identification and introjects are precursors of the process of identity formation in adolescence, and their mastery in childhood paves the way for adolescents to have greater success in mastering the developmental demands they face, which include adapting to significantly stronger and more diverse instinctual impulses and bidding farewell, often sadly, to the self and objects of childhood (Jacobson 1964).

# Developmental Aspects of Identity in Adolescence

Erikson (1968) posited that identity formation occurs as the adolescent begins to selectively retain and relinquish the identifications of childhood, which are no longer seen as useful. By late adolescence, adolescents describe their goals without indicating the source, be it parents, other role models, or objects of identification (Harter 2012). It is as if these older adolescents "own these various choices" after having selected among the "self-guides…

[which are] increasingly internalized and less tied to their social origins" (Harter 2008, p. 246). Family, peers, and the community react to the new self that is beginning to form. Erikson describes the mutuality in this process: "the community feels recognized by the individual who cares to ask for recognition...and can feel deeply—and vengefully—rejected by the individual who does not seem to care" (Erikson 1968, p. 160). Thus, the stakes are high between adolescent and parent, as each needs to feel meaningful in the eyes of the other. For the adolescent, it is crucial that they not feel forced to make a premature commitment to satisfy parents or other adults, lest they experience a sense of shame or feel shamed in the eyes of their peers. For Erikson, the concept of "crisis" in this process signifies a "turning point, a crucial period of increased vulnerability and heightened potential" (Erikson 1968, p. 96), and the designation of an identity crisis in an adolescent usually signifies that those who are important in his or her life do not offer confirmation of this changing identity as being meaningful, or as making sense in terms of who the adolescent was and where he or she is going. This may often occur when the parents feel that the course their child is taking invalidates how they have seen themselves as parents. Therefore, the identities of both parent and adolescent are felt to be at stake. But, with a supportive moratorium period, the adolescent can experiment and try out different roles without the fear that premature commitments will be demanded of him or her, and parents can minimize their worry about being abandoned or rejected.

## Case 2: Joe

Joe, a 20-years-old, first began psychotherapy in middle school because his learning problems contributed to anxiety, procrastination, or outright refusal to do work. Psychotherapy was discontinued by the second year of high school, at which time he was functioning quite well, but was resumed after he dropped out during his third year of college. Although he obtained very satisfactory grades during his first year at a demanding college, he began procrastinating again, fell too far behind to catch up, and left college to return to live at home. Although Joe was no longer in adolescence, his struggle is informative about what can occur when the desired integration of identity elements does not occur. Once back at home, he did not readily seek a job or resume college. He was a good family member, often taking care of the house and shopping and cooking for everyone. In therapy he realized that he did not know what he wanted to do, and he stopped working at college when commitment to a major was demanded. His parents were good, caring people who were successful and hardworking. His avoidance of work, of "taking care of business," made them anxious for him, often presented in reaction to his omnipotent control and frequent lying. His father would frequently ask Joe about his plan because that was how his father approached life and dealt with anxiety, but Joe was totally puzzled by the question and the orientation it represented. Their heated arguments were in service of each maintaining a view of self and the world.

# Identity Diffusion Versus Identity Crisis

Normal adolescence may sometimes be difficult to distinguish from more pathological elements. BPD symptoms appear to peak from 14 to 17 years of age and then begin to decline (Bornovalova et al. 2009). It may be that this pattern is attributable to developmental changes in brain structures, with the decline in BPD symptoms associated with developing control mechanisms coming online (Powers and Casey 2015). It is also interesting to consider the possible contribution of the development of abstract thinking during adolescence, which of course is also subject to neurodevelopmental and genetic contributions.

When individuals are asked to describe themselves, they typically offer several attributes, characteristics they show in particular situations (e.g., how they would describe themselves when with close friends and how they see themselves when they are in a larger peer group). Harter (2008), in reviewing research by neo-Piagetians, indicates that in early adolescence the youngster tends to offer individual, isolated descriptors (e.g., "I am friendly"). However, the growth in abstract thinking in middle adolescence may promote simultaneous comparisons between descriptors. These comparisons can often involve linking opposite attributes, leading to unstable self-representations and confusion, and raising tension about "who am I, really?" (e.g., "Am I really fun and friendly? [like I am with my closest friends] or am I quiet and withdrawn [like I am in a large group]?"; "How come my mood switches from being happy when I'm with my friends to being anxious and nasty with my parents when I get home?"). Girls at this age were found to be more sensitive to these contradictions than boys. Harter (2008) posits that these mid-adolescents want to create a coherent, uniform representation of their self but may not be able to generate the more abstract, higher-order concepts that allow for this. It is only in late adolescence that they have the cognitive wherewithal to generate representations that integrate these individual, contradictory descriptors. Higher-order concepts (e.g., "I am flexible, adaptive, moody") provide a way to create a more integrated, coherent self-image across time and situation. Therefore, as noted in Chapter 1, we might expect that for those who show a continuance of BPD symptoms, for whom it is not a stage-specific phenomenon (cf. Moffitt 1993a), more is involved than the contribution of advanced abstract thinking, and the crisis is not normative. In the normative condition, it is less likely that PD features such as true splitting would be seen.

Marcia (Kroger and Marcia 2011; Kroger et al. 2010) suggests in the Erikson-Marcia tradition that the intersection of the processes of Exploration (referred to as "Crisis" in his earlier writing) and Commitment can describe the course of identity formation. Exploration involves experimenting with different roles and plans in order to select among meaningful options. Commitment reflects the degree of investment in a course of action or belief. He developed the Identity Status Interview (Marcia and Archer 1993) to ask how individuals arrived at their commitments while examining the areas of occupational and ideological (e.g., religion, politics) choice. The status of High Commitment includes those with Identity Achieved status, who arrived at their commitments after engaging in Exploration, and those with a Foreclosure status, who experienced minimal evaluation and basically acquired their commitments from others or had it "conferred" on them. Foreclosed individuals tend to be brittle or fragile and defensive in maintaining their position and might include individuals with narcissistic PD. The status of Low Commitment includes individuals with Moratorium status, who are engaging in exploration and may be struggling to reach commitment but are moving forward, and others who are more inclined to ruminate and freeze. The status of Identity Diffusion includes individuals who are uncommitted and show little exploration. These may be individuals who are easily swayed, show the lowest level of secure attachment, may also have been characterized by avoidant attachments, and have low levels of parental acceptance. Marcia and colleagues' research showed that Identity Achieved individuals have the highest level of secure attachment. There is also a Reconsideration process that promotes a review of commitments. If commitments are weakened, increased anxiety can be expected because some may feel role confusion, worries about not working enough toward being something, or renewed fear of premature commitment.

The usefulness of these categories for the clinician may be that inquiries about the joint processes of commitment and exploration can help in diagnosing, understanding, and treating the adolescent. Normal adolescent development in Western society can be viewed as a time of exploration and normative crises. Just as parental reactions were important in mirroring the early phases of childhood self and object formation, here too the parents' ability to be empathic while differentiating themselves from their adolescent's needs and anxieties becomes important. Consider once again the case of Joe, the 20-year-old introduced earlier:

## Case 2: Joe (*continued*)

Aside from the general role that anxiety was playing in Joe's life, his fear of making a commitment to a major that he was uncertain about, that he "sort of just fell into," led him to withdraw from working at his courses. Although he was receiving a failing grade in most courses in his second year, he could not tell or disappoint his academically and professionally successful parents, whom he cared about. The issue of commitment touched on other aspects of his life, such as emotional and sexual intimacy. His time living at home became more pleasant for him and his parents once he came to recognize and understand his anxiety about commitment (be it premature or inauthentic commitment), and he then found a way to explain himself to his parents so that they could understand and be more accepting of the direction he was going at that time. They still experienced an appropriate or understandable level of anxiety about his future, but they realized he was trying even though he appeared "stuck." He was also "stuck" because of a defensive structure that prevented him from experiencing most feelings other than anger.

# Summary

When the developmental stage of normal identity integration is not reached (when there is an absence of integrated concepts of self and other), the earlier developmental stage of dissociation or splitting between an idealized and a persecutory segment of experience persists. Under these conditions, multiple, nonintegrated representations of self split into an idealized and a persecutory segment, and multiple representations of significant others split along similar lines, jointly constituting the syndrome of identity diffusion. One central consequence of identity diffusion is the incapacity under the influence of a peak affect state to assess that affect state from the perspective of an integrated sense of self. The particular mental state may be fully experienced in consciousness but cannot be put into the context of one's total self experience, implying a serious loss of the normal capacity for self-reflection—that is, for mentalization—and with this, balanced and integrated representations of self and other are not possible. In brief, the subjective experience of a person with a split psychological structure is that the person is what he or she feels in any given moment, totally disconnected from what he or she may feel at another moment. TFP-A, when interpreting splitting and other primitive defensive operations, fosters mentalization by creating a set of conditions that promotes the integration of these conscious but contradictory and disconnected representations of self and other. The development of an integrated representation of self facilitates the self-reflective function regarding the particular peak mental state under consideration. Thus, starting from a temperamental predisposition marked by a predominance of negative affect and impulsivity, and deficits in effortful control, the development of disorganized attachment, exposure to physical or sexual trauma, abandonment, or chronic family chaos predisposes the individual to pathological fixation at an early stage of development that predates the integration of normal identity. A general split then persists between the idealized and persecutory internalized experiences under the dominance of corresponding negative and positive peak affect states.

Clinically, identity diffusion accounts for the defining characteristics of borderline personality organization. The predominance of primitive dissociation or splitting of the idealized segment of experience from the paranoid one is reinforced by primitive defensive operations intimately connected with splitting mechanisms, such as projective identification, denial, primitive idealization, devaluation, omnipotence, and omnipotent control. All these defensive mechanisms contribute to distorting interpersonal interactions and create chronic disturbances in interpersonal relationships, thus reinforcing the lack of self-reflectiveness and of "mentalization" in a broad sense, decreasing the capacity to assess other people's behavior and motivation in depth, particularly, of course, under the effect of intense affect activation. So too is there interference with a comprehensive integration of one's past and present into a capacity to predict one's future behavior and a decrease in the capacity for stable commitment to professional goals, personal interests, work and social functions, and intimate relationships.

# PART II

Therapeutic Approach

# CHAPTER 3

# Major Goal and Strategies

**THE MAIN GOAL** of Transference-Focused Psychotherapy for Adolescents (TFP-A) is *identity integration*—that is, the integration of mutually split-off idealized and persecutory internalized object relations that surface in the transference in order to achieve a coherent, realistic, and stable experience of self and others as well as to face developmental endeavors. Achieving this goal should modify the disabling personality structure, and thus the course of personality development, sufficiently to meaningfully improve functioning in the realms of studies and work, professional choices, and intimate relations.

To achieve this goal clinically, we outline a number of generally sequential steps, the strategies of TFP-A, in which the goal is to integrate part-self and part-object representations through a process by which underlying representations are recognized and marked by the therapist and then delineated as characteristic patterns of experiencing, relating, or disrupting the developmental challenges. The treatment strategies pertain to the long-term objectives of the treatment and are geared toward the integration of the adolescent split-off internalized self and other representations. They are basically guidelines for staying focused on the main task of working on the adolescent's internal world even when the therapy session or the adolescent's external life is chaotic.

The main strategy of TFP-A consists in the facilitation of the (re)activation in the treatment of split-off internalized object relations of contrasting persecutory and idealized nature that are observed and interpreted in the transference. As in the adult treatment, the adolescent is instructed to carry out free association. The therapist restricts his or her role to careful observation of the activation of regressive, split-off relations in the transference, to help the adolescent to identify them, and to interpret their segregation in

49

the light of the adolescent's enormous difficulty in reflecting on his of her own behavior and on the interactions the adolescent gets involved in.

The interpretation of these split-off object relations is based on the assumption that each of them reflects a dyadic unit of a self representation, an object representation, and a dominant affect linking them, and that the activation of these dyadic relationships determines the adolescent's perception of the therapist and entails rapid role reversals in the transference: the adolescent may identify with a primitive self representation while projecting a corresponding object representation onto the therapist, but 10 minutes later, the adolescent may identify with the object representation while projecting the self representation onto the therapist. Engaging the adolescent's observing ego in this phenomenon paves the way for interpreting the conflicts that keep these dyads, and the corresponding views of self and other, separate and exaggerated. For example, the adolescent might present himself as the victim, who is taken advantage of, abused, ignored, degraded, or made to feel insignificant (i.e, victimized) by family, friend, or therapist (i.e., the victimizer), yet a short while later may become critical or ignoring or demeaning toward the therapist (i.e., now the adolescent becomes the victimizer and the therapist is the victim). Until these representations are integrated into more nuanced and modulated ones, the adolescent will continue to perceive himself and others in exaggerated, distorted, and rapidly shifting terms. The oscillation or alternative distribution of the roles of each dyad has to be differentiated from the fundamental split between opposite dyads carrying opposite (idealizing and persecutory) affective charges.[1]

The final step of interpretation consists in the linking of the dissociated positive and negative transferences, leading to an integration of the mutually split-off idealized and persecutory segments of experience with the corresponding resolution of identity diffusion. The interpretation of these split-off relationships occurs in a characteristic sequence of three steps:

1. Description of the total relationship that seems to be activated at that point, using metaphorical statements to present the situation as completely as possible in a way that can be understood by the adolescent, and

---

[1]Most students learning Transference-Focused Psychotherapy (TFP) have a hard time understanding the difference between role reversals within the dyad and the split between opposing dyads—they think "the victim is the good object and the aggressor is the bad object." We have to remind them that being a victim isn't really good.

the clarification of who enacts what role in that interaction. The therapist's comments are based on his or her observations and countertransference[2] utilization, and on clarifications[3] that have been sought of the adolescent's experience of the relationship at each moment.

2. Observation of the interchange of the corresponding roles between patient and therapist, an extremely important step that permits the adolescent, throughout time, to understand her unconscious identification with the object representation as well as with the self representation, leading to a gradual awareness of the mutual complementarity of these two roles. This second step is carried out in the clarification and confrontation[4] of both of the oscillating poles of a given dyad. However, since the idealized and persecutory relationships that are activated remain typically split-off from each other in different dyads, the patient becomes more able to recognize the extreme dyadic nature of each of them while still maintaining the split or dissociated nature that separates "all good" from "all bad" relationships. Understanding the motivation for keeping these dyads separate is one of the main objectives of the interpretative work, the focus of the next step.

3. Interpretative linking of the mutually dissociated positive and negative transferences, the transferences reflecting the idealized and persecutory relationships, thus leading to an integration of the mutually split-off idealized and persecutory segments of experience, the corresponding resolution of identity diffusion, and the modulation of intense affect dispositions as primitive euphoric or hypomanic affects are integrated with their corresponding fearful, persecutory, and aggressive opposites. This third step brings about a significant integration of the patient's ego identity, as an integrated view of self—more complex, rich, and nuanced than the simplistic and extreme split-off self representations—and a corre-

---

[2]Countertransference is defined as the "provoked and expected reactions" induced in the therapist by the patient's transference. It is used to evaluate the degree of regression in the patient and to identify the part of the patient's experience that is split-off and projected in the therapist. Unaware countertransference may challenge the therapist's identity, equilibrium, and neutrality.

[3]Clarification usually involves the therapist's asking the patient for more detail to fill out the gaps until the complete picture emerges and then elaborating, clarifying the links, reordering, and restating the material in the service of fully understanding and appreciating the patient's experience.

[4]Confrontation is used to bring to the person's awareness contradiction of affects, representations, and conflicts.

sponding integrated view of significant others replace their split-off previous nature. An experience of appropriate depressive affects, reflecting the capacity for acknowledging one's own aggression that had previously been projected or experienced as dysphoric affect, with the emergence of concern, guilt, and the wish to repair good relationships damaged in fantasy or reality by the individual's previously denied and projected aggressive affects, becomes dominant. The integration of mutually split-off idealized and persecutory representation of self and of corresponding idealized and persecutory representations of significant others also brings about the mutual penetration and toning down of extreme, opposite affect states linked to these representations. This modulation of affective experiences facilitates affect regulation, an increased capacity for affect control, by the strengthening of their cognitive context as a consequence of the integration of self and object representations. Significative increase in cognitive framing of affective states, in short, improves mentalization—that is, the capacity for realistic assessment of mental states of self and significant others—together with impulse control and enrichment of the overall subtlety and complexity of the assessment of social interactions.

The first step of this sequence begins in the first therapy session, and the second step follows relatively quickly after the first few weeks and months of treatment. The third step characterizes the middle and advanced stages of the psychotherapy. At the same time, however, this three-step sequence is a highly recursive process. Some interpretations that occur at the third step may become possible relatively early, and the three steps may recycle again and again, with the entire sequence first taking weeks to develop and then taking place over the course of a few sessions. In the advanced stages of the treatment, all three steps eventually may be elaborated in the course of the same session.

In the early stages of the treatment there may be a strong affective dominance of an adolescent's communication about his or her relations with significant others in the external world. This reflects both the predominance of acting out and splitting mechanisms, as well as the frequent, significant difficulties that adolescents with borderline personality disorder have in reflecting on their emotional experiences in the therapeutic hours. They may present little tolerance for direct analysis of their relationship with the therapist and may split off manifest positive transference reactions in the hours from the acting out of negative transferences with other objects, and by means of somatization. The therapist's analysis of the emotional implications of those external relations prepares the road to transference analysis in a later stage of the treatment. The utilization of the adolescent's own metaphors in the description of his or her conflicts outside the therapeutic hours may serve as bridging concepts for transference analysis.

Stereotypical defensive distortions of the therapist's personality and interventions as perceived by the patient, in terms of the corresponding adolescent cultural stereotypes, may need to be made explicit and gradually worked through before deeper and more significant transference developments can be interpreted. The stereotype includes the therapist as "agent" of the parents, as "unknown and dangerous" adult, and as seductive and frightening hypocrite, and the therapist's tolerance may be interpreted as weakness or stupidity.

In general, the strategic steps of TFP-A evolve slowly, with much more time required to explore and clarify the interchange between self and object representations in the transference, and a correspondingly slower rate of working through of primitive defensive operations in the transference. This process is encouraged by helping the adolescent to develop a curiosity and marked interest in his or her own hypothesis.

The careful exploration of the patient's perceptions of significant others—helping the patient to reflect on why other people may react the way they do and on how the patient's reactions to the perceived behavior of others can be understood and verbalized—provides important preparatory material for the interpretation of projective identification[5] and acting out[6] in the transference.

Tolerant exploration of the significance of transference developments, particularly of the acting out of negative transferences in the therapeutic hours, including a "detoxifying," "playful" exploring of the fantasy implications of transferential acting out, provides an important space for enactment and gradual interpretative resolution of dominant transferences and of the sharp splitting between idealizing and paranoid transferences toward the therapist.

The potential for serious transference acting out, reflected in missing sessions, general efforts to interrupt the therapy on the part of the patient, and provocative behavior at home geared to pit therapist and parents

---

[5]Projective identification is an attempt to make the other (the therapist) feel unbearable thoughts or feelings that cannot be tolerated in the self.
[6]Acting out in the transference is the direct expression of conflicts in the here and now in preference to reflecting on them.

against each other, needs to be addressed in the sessions. If attempts to do this are unsuccessful, the therapist prioritizes maintenance of the structure and frame of the treatment. Meetings with parents may be necessary to deal with adolescent acting out or the emotional reactions of the adolescent and parents.

Perhaps the greatest difficulty in deepening the strategic analysis of dominant idealized and persecutory relationships and their mutual dissociation in the transference is presented by adolescents with narcissistic personality disorder, particularly those with the frequently present tendency toward antisocial behavior. When significant antisocial behavior threatens the adolescent with expulsion from school or involvement in legal procedures, a clear structuring and controlled setting on the part of home and school may be an indispensable correlate of the possibility of exploring the corresponding conflicts in the treatment. The therapist, as always, has to be "moral but not moralistic" and explore the dynamics of the antisocial behavior and, particularly, the related self-destructive risks. When, on the other hand, an excessively severe and even sadistic "clamping down" on an adolescent's behavior evolves on the part of parents, school, or other authorities, the therapist taking a stand in terms of what would seem realistic expectations of him may only seemingly signify an abandonment of technical neutrality.[7]

In the case of narcissistic pathology without significant antisocial behavior but with the characteristic activation of an omnipotent, devaluing pathological grandiose self in the transference, and acting out of self-destructive grandiosity at home, on the street, and at school, the relation between the pathological grandiose self and the split-off, devalued, humiliated part of the self of the patient may determine a dominant negative transference pattern over an extended period of time, with only very gradual emergence of the capacity for normal dependence in the transference. Here the strategic objective of the treatment may, for a long time, be limited to the gradual dismantling of that pathological grandiose self to reveal the underlying disarray, fragmentation, and confusion that had been, up to that point, defensively kept out of awareness by the consistent devaluing grandiosity.

In some cases, the presence of secondary gain of illness complicates the treatment situation, aggravating the prognosis and requiring the collaboration of parents and school in sustaining the structure of the treatment. This

---

[7]Technical neutrality is a therapeutic stance in which the therapist stays neutral and nonjudgmental in the face of opposite sides of an adolescent conflict.

situation involves the negotiation of a treatment contract, which will be discussed in Chapter 5 of this manual. For example, adolescents who get "too anxious" to go to school but are perfectly happy partying with their friends may represent such a situation; in other cases, a prevailing general passivity and efforts to obtain privileges "because of emotional difficulties" provide an adolescent with the motivation to hold on to symptoms and difficulties. Here, the therapist's support of an appropriate control of the structure and conditions of the treatment by the parents is appropriate, as long as such conditions for treatment are spelled out patiently in combined adolescent-parent-therapist sessions and the patient's transference reaction to the therapist's intervention is fully explored.

When severe identity diffusion and the corresponding splitting in transference developments are gradually overcome, the sessions may become more differentiated in their emotional implications, and acting out should decrease. Severe turmoil in the sessions while the external life of the adolescent normalizes is a good indicator of progress in the strategic efforts of the therapist.

# CHAPTER 4

# Clinical Evaluation and Assessment Process

**THE ASSESSMENT PHASE** in Transference-Focused Psychotherapy for Adolescents (TFP-A) establishes and adheres to a process that quickly incorporates many elements that will define the role of each participant in both the assessment phase and throughout the treatment itself, should TFP-A be the recommended treatment of choice. Additionally, the Transference-Focused Psychotherapy (TFP) techniques that are relied on in the treatment, such as clarification, confrontation, and use of transference and countertransference information, as well as the maintenance of technical neutrality, are employed in the assessment interview. These techniques will be described in greater detail in Chapter 6.

The following features of the TFP-A assessment process will be described in this chapter:

1. Adherence to procedures even in the face of possible extenuating circumstances.
2. Explanation of the evaluation process to the adolescent and his or her parents.
3. Comprehensive diagnostic procedures that examine the adolescent's range of current functioning, including psychopathology viewed broadly, with a consideration of dysfunction of mood, behavior, and thought, guided or informed by a variety of procedures. We will pay particular attention to constructs and procedures that derive from the TFP model so that we can focus on the adolescent's current personality organization and its ramifications.
4. Examination of parental functioning to get a sense of parents' contribution to the development and maintenance of the adolescent's current status and to determine their ability to cooperate with and support the TFP-

A psychotherapy process. The information obtained when carrying out items 3 and 4 contributes to an analysis of questions of comorbidity and the differential diagnosis of the adolescent's presenting problems. This is necessary for determining whether TFP-A is the recommended treatment of choice.

5. Presentation to the adolescent and parents of the findings of the evaluation.

# Initiation of the Evaluation and Procedural Adherence

The opening of the assessment phase provides the initial contact with the adolescent and his or her family, and so, from the very start, factors that contribute to establishing the treatment frame are present. For example, if the adolescent and the family present in crisis, the crisis is dealt with (e.g., emergency room visit; serious drug problem), and only after safety and order are established, which could even require a period of time in another form of treatment (e.g., addiction program; eating disorders program), can in-depth evaluation and treatment planning proceed. Thus, the role of the evaluation process does not get circumvented or replaced by a rush to begin psychotherapy, especially in the face of crisis.

A presenting initial crisis immediately calls into play some of the fundamental TFP-A tools. The sense of emergency that is likely to be experienced by the parents can induce countertransference that may include a contagious sense of urgency to do something either to calm the parents or to obtain their approval. The therapist is thereby unconsciously drawn into the family system in which the adolescent may feel overlooked or ignored because the therapist, perhaps unconsciously identifying with the adolescent, turns to taking care of the parents so as to promote their adequacy as parents. Alternatively, the therapist may feel a pull to save the adolescent and thus become part of a different dyad in which the therapist becomes the "good parent" who rescues the needy, failing child from her inadequate parents. Thus, the importance of maintaining technical neutrality should be kept in mind even at the very beginning of the assessment.

## Case 1: Anna

Anna, a 19-year-old with previous diagnoses of borderline personality disorder (BPD), narcissistic personality disorder (PD), and antisocial PD, was being evaluated. Despite 3 years of various attempts at treatment, including residential treatment programs, hospitalizations, and attempts at outpatient psychotherapy, her current situation was untenable, and therapy was not proving effective and was poorly attended. Anna did not appear at her first scheduled meeting with parents and the consulting therapist, but she attended the second scheduled meeting and seemed engaged in both individual and parental components of this prolonged meeting. However, she did not appear at her next scheduled individual meeting, consistent with her previous patterns of engagement. Her mother sent a message warning the therapist that Anna might not attend this meeting, and when the therapist contacted Anna merely to confirm their appointment, she replied, "I bet my mother told you to do this." The mother, meanwhile, sent an additional message expressing a wish to talk to the therapist again before another meeting was held with Anna, if one were to occur. This request did not have the quality of an emergency contact. Therefore, the therapist was immediately placed between the mother and daughter in their struggle (which reflected their issues over attachment and separation), and the countertransference included strong discomfort and a sense of being controlled and directed, and a feeling that if one party was to be satisfied, the other would feel angry, hurt, and rejected and might flee therapy. Thus, the assessment itself felt in jeopardy from the very beginning.

The therapist attempted to maintain neutrality by emphasizing the need to adhere to the process as originally explained, with its objective of completing an evaluation and providing a recommendation. It is also valuable for the therapist to keep in mind who is the patient (i.e., the adolescent) and who is the one to whom the therapist is being pulled to respond. To this end, in the case of Anna, the consultation proceeded as originally planned without calling her mother, but the therapist explained to parent and adolescent that the initial plan agreed to in the first session would be adhered to and a meeting would be scheduled with the adolescent as planned without diverting to other demands that each was making on the therapist. It was explained that this was thought to be the best way to maintain the process and not get derailed by the types of demands and conflicts each party had described in that first session that contributed to why they needed to seek this consultation in the first place.

As will be seen, this approach in the assessment phase adheres to concepts that inform the contract phase and its implementation, to be described in Chapter 5.

# Rationale for the Evaluation Process

Evaluation according to the TFP-A model involves a comprehensive diagnostic assessment that seeks to obtain a clear picture of the adolescent's current level of personality development and to determine if any other features of psychopathology are contributing to the behaviors that prompted the adolescent and his or her family to seek help. A principal goal is to get a relatively complete picture of the adolescent's overall level of functioning, including his or her personality organization, and to distinguish between the normal identity confusion (crisis) that is commonly encountered at adolescence, for which a less intensive intervention may be sufficient, and the identity diffusion that underlies PDs, for which TFP-A treatment is particularly well suited. These various goals are approached with an initial meeting with parents and adolescent, separate meetings with parents and with adolescent, and a joint meeting to discuss findings and recommendations. The number of meetings of each type varies with the each case's level of complexity. The rationale and execution for this approach, as well as exceptions to this model, will be described at different points in this chapter.

A comprehensive evaluation is necessary because adolescent PDs are associated with high comorbidity, especially mood disorders, as well as with anxiety, behavioral, and attention-deficit disorders (Shiner and Allen 2013). While there may be debate about how best to understand this comorbidity, it is indisputable that adolescent PDs can be embedded in a complex network of difficulties that can mask the PD and mislead the clinician. Therefore, the clinician needs a clear picture of the adolescent's full range of functioning in order to arrive at an understanding of the contribution of personality problems to his/her overall problems. For example, many adolescents experience a mixed course following a diagnosis and treatment for depression. Because adolescents with BPD may complain of depressed mood, report irritability, and describe a quality of anhedonia (which may actually be more akin to the feeling of emptiness associated with BPD), it is not surprising that some of these youngsters will be treated for depression but show minimal improvement. Added confusion may arise because many adolescents are not particularly responsive to antidepressant medication (Hammad et al. 2006; Paton et al. 2015), leaving some clinicians and psychiatrists wondering if there may be another contributing factor, such as a psychotic process, that requires a different class of medication. Therefore, an awareness of how to unpack this complex picture and identify and treat PDs in adolescence is very important lest the effective treatment of the mood, anxiety, and disruptive or impulse-control disorders also be undermined. This situation may occur with greater frequency than anticipated because although most clinicians who work with young people acknowledge that BPD can be diagnosed in adolescence, a relatively small percentage actually do so (Laurenssen et al. 2013).

Typically, the adolescent and parents do not present for therapy saying that they think he or she may have a PD, although there is a somewhat greater awareness of borderline and narcissistic PDs than in the past. Instead, they will describe concerns about anxiety, mood, anger, or interpersonal functioning with family, peers, and school. The clinician's task is to explain the TFP-A assessment process to the adolescent and parents so that they can appreciate the relationship between this process and their concerns that brought them. This discussion will focus on the purpose of assessment, including the need to understand the nature of the adolescent's problems, culminating in a determination of an appropriate treatment choice. The adolescent and parents are told that it will take at least several sessions for the assessment to be completed. This process will culminate in feedback that will lead to an explanation of the findings, treatment recommendation(s), and, if TFP-A is recommended, formulation of a treatment contract (see Chapter 5). This is an agreement that will outline the responsibilities and expectations for the clinician, the adolescent, and the parents, including a strategy for addressing immediate and long-term emergencies. This process helps preserve the integrity and viability of the treatment. Thus, from the very first contact through the feedback meeting, before psychotherapy proper has begun, the clinician's actions promote the establishment of a relationship with the adolescent so that the clinician can be seen as curious, serious, interested, and competent, with an empathic understanding of the adolescent, while not conveying a quality of intimacy or closeness that fosters dependency or engenders in the adolescent concerns about regressive pulls.

# Presentation of the Evaluation Process

## Opening Considerations, Explanations, and Explorations With Adolescent and Parents

In order for the adolescent and the parents to appreciate the evaluation process, the TFP-A therapist may provide a layperson's explanation of the complexity behind the problems in young people that necessitate such a comprehensive evaluation. It is then understandable that the evaluation will take several meetings, after which the therapist's impressions and recommendations will be offered. Our typical format is to meet first with the parents and adolescent, then with the adolescent alone and the parents alone, and hold a feedback meeting with the adolescent and parents. It can be necessary to have several meetings with just the adolescent in order to obtain a clear picture of his or her level of personality organization. The rationale for this sequence follows.

It can be a dilemma for therapists to decide how to initiate the interviewing process when an adolescent is the identified patient. Should they meet first with the adolescent alone, with the parents alone, or with all of them? The adolescent can be seen as having the right to come alone, and many feel that doing so sends a clear message to all parties that confidentiality and respect for the developing autonomy of the adolescent are being supported. But it is still apparent to everyone that the adolescent remains under the parent's responsibility and authority, and the therapist needs to help all parties clarify their roles, often over time, to support the therapy and, in so doing, support the adolescent's movement toward a healthier developmental trajectory.

The complicated struggle that can occur over the issues of responsibility and autonomy can become extreme, impacting even the initiation of the therapy as well as the therapy itself, and is a theme that may be expressed somewhat differently with older than with younger adolescents. For example, some adolescents, to their detriment, exercise omnipotent control and defeat the parents and make them feel helpless; as a result the situation may not improve or may deteriorate over time. The parents remain in this helpless mode and find themselves unable to consistently establish and follow through on their previous demands or on agreements reached with the adolescent, including those that were developed with the help of prior consultations. After the parents and consultants are then stymied, the parents may struggle further to follow ensuing suggestions to accept limitations on what they might accomplish and to let their child "sink or swim." Understandably, their guilt, fear, anger, and anxiety can be considerable.

Anna, the 19-year-old described earlier, had a lifestyle that maintained a maladaptive, potentially dangerous, and complicated status quo with her parents because, despite her grandiose protestations about not being able to tolerate being with her parents, she also reversed roles and expressed another aspect of the dyad by indicating that she would like to be able to live at home. Her noncompliance and seemingly deliberate oppositional behavior made this impossible but allowed her to say to the TFP-A consultant that "they would not let me live at home," portraying herself as the rejected, unwanted victim. In effect, she alternated between the roles of the defiant, pseudo-independent one who had all the power, and the frightened one who still needed care and could not effectively step out into the world. Her anger and especially her anxiety were successfully projected onto her parents. Thus, their joint attachment problems, anxiety, hostility, and guilt prevented movement forward.

In a situation like Anna's, parents may still feel some need to take care of their child and so cannot readily reject him or her—and neither their child nor their social network often expects this of them despite sometimes advising them to. In effect, even when there is significant conflict and push for separation, parents typically face the pressure to be responsible and do something and may be drawn into applying counter-controlling methods, keeping them very much involved in their child's life. Our approach to treatment tries to recognize this by initially involving the parents in collaboration toward the goals of furthering and supporting a healthy separation process as part of the therapy process. This collaborative approach is reflected in the assessment phase by recognizing and even supporting the reality of the parents' role and their responsibility, while also respecting and encouraging the adolescent's autonomy when expressed in adaptive, growth-producing ways.

With other parenting situations, particularly neglectful ones, the clinician may find it necessary to do preliminary work to determine the level of commitment and responsibility the parents are able or willing to take on and to work at preparing them to assume a stance that would be supportive of the therapy and maintain appropriate boundaries with their child. When parents are not able to take on such responsibility, which typically extends well beyond the therapy itself, but allow for therapy to proceed, the treatment can include helping the adolescent to learn to recognize and accept their parents' limitations and to distinguish himself or herself from the parents' hostile, rejecting, or ignoring style.

These sorts of complicated relationship patterns that may be seen in the lives of adolescents with severe, enduring problems that often characterize those with PD lead us to prefer meeting first with the adolescent and their parents. This preference offers an initial perspective that the therapist is interested in seeing how the family works, from the beginning, and that all the members can make an important contribution to the therapist's understanding of the "story" of this adolescent and the family as the therapist continues to pursue an understanding of the adolescent's individual and personality difficulties. The therapist should clearly distinguish these meetings from therapy proper while asserting that it is an important first step in identifying problems and goals and for determining what the therapist will recommend as a plan of action. Even when an adolescent seems engaged and responsive in this first joint meeting, the therapist reminds all parties that the adolescent will have his or her own meetings with the therapist and that "in our meetings you can talk about your personal views as well as your views about their understanding of you and your family." (The interviewing techniques used in the individual meeting with the adolescent will be described later in this chapter.) The therapist can also present a summary of what he or she learned during this meeting, ask the others about what they learned, and ask the adolescent "if you wish to comment" on these perceptions.

A separate meeting with parents is also held. This contributes toward the assessment of developmental issues and is essential for obtaining a picture of the adolescent's premorbid level of functioning. An awareness of the adolescent's highest level of premorbid functioning, the possibility of a downward inflection point in his or her development, the age at which it occurred, and concurrent events that may have been precipitants are best provided by the parents; all this information provides a frame of reference for a deeper understanding of the present situation, especially when the adolescent presents in crisis.

The clinician, through his or her questioning, attempts to move the parents from a description of current symptoms and developmental "facts" through their understanding or hypotheses about what motivates their child. This process also provides a sense of their ability to take their child's perspective and their mentalizing capacity. The parent meeting may also increase parents' awareness that they can help the clinician understand the adolescent and his or her impact on the family, and that they play an important role in helping the assessment and the therapy itself. The clinician begins to determine whether the parents will be able to collaborate. Or will they interfere? Can they tolerate anxiety and be helpful, or will they become overwrought by anxiety and undermine the implementation of contractual plans? By providing insight into each parent's identity and interpersonal functioning, the parent meetings also help the clinician to determine if attempting to make a change in parental functioning is indicated or possible—will it be possible to count on the parent to change and to tolerate and support change? For example, in Anna's situation, it was discovered that her mother became a container for her anxiety and Anna did not face demands and expectations to learn how to experience or take ownership of her anxiety, so she never really learned how to modulate the anxiety and master the situations that promoted it. As a result, the consultant made sure to ask Anna, "Tell me about what it is like for you to get anxious," and she replied, "I don't do anxiety well!" Consistent with the dyads and interactional patterns described here, she then subtly moved to change the topic. The formation of the clinician's insights and the nature of the questioning of Anna were informed by having the parent meeting and allowed for the consideration of additional important diagnostic questions, such as the presence of projective identification or enmeshed attachment patterns, that could help in understanding the nature of experienced anxiety in this family.

# The Resistant Adolescent

An alternative pathway becomes necessary with those adolescents who present with an aggressive stance and extreme resistance to the treatment. They often require an initial individual meeting, separate from the type of semi-structured diagnostic interviewing to be described later in this chapter, to try to get the assessment on track. The clinician will acknowledge the adolescent's resistance and might consider pointing out that they (adolescent and clinician) "are stuck and share a problem." The parents are asking the clinician to help all of them, and they are also asking the adolescent to behave/conform and so forth. Therefore, the parents want both the therapist and the adolescent to give something so that perhaps they can come to an understanding of what can be given to the parents and what the adolescent can receive and profit from during this process without compromising what the adolescent feels is important to his or her sense of self. In effect, the adolescent can be helped to realize he or she is in a powerful position and can stymie the clinician as he or she has done with the parents. "So you have defeated me! You have another notch on your belt! But I'm interested in learning from you where that leaves you." If the adolescent is so intent on not giving to the parents, then the clinician will not be able to either. But, the clinician can broaden the adolescent's awareness and move the focus from a single entity (either the adolescent himself or herself *or* the parent) to a dual, more complex focus: "If I cannot give anything to your parents, then I may not be able to give anything to you, and if you deny them, you end up denying yourself. So let's distinguish your struggle with them from how it creates a struggle within your self." Fostering this type of awareness begins the process of movement toward mutuality and interdependency that promotes growth and creates realistic and useful dyads. Anna, the 19-year-old discussed earlier, after an initial moment of confusion and disbelief, was shocked to realize that while she overtly expressed a sense of powerlessness and victimization, she was actually very powerful and controlling of her mother's emotions and some of her actions.

A minimal goal with some of these resistant adolescents could be to do an assessment that leads to a recommendation. The clinician should emphasize to both adolescent and parents that the purpose of the evaluation process is to decide if treatment, at least of the TFP-A variety, is appropriate. Thus, in some situations there could be a suggestion of no treatment—a statement that therapy at this time may not be the best decision, despite what the parents believe and hope for.

It may be difficult for the adolescent to believe that the clinician could be objective, to not automatically be on the parents' side. But it is possible that the parents' expectation is not in accord with what the adolescent wants or needs. However, in order to expand the conversation and the adolescent's range of thinking—the clinician can ask whether the adolescent would be willing to consider the possibility that his or her discussions with the clinician could give rise to objectives and goals that the adolescent may desire, resulting in a wish for change that is independent of what parents or school may desire. "It's understandable that you would not want to participate in a process that you feel doesn't give you something." Indeed, the clinician can convey his or her hesitancy about moving ahead if the adolescent cannot develop desirable personal goals. Without them, "Why would you want to participate?" and "I would be uneasy." Thus, for the clinician, a goal would be for the adolescent to come to understand that his or her objectives might be separate and distinct from those of the parents. By moving the focus from the parents' wishes (demands, as viewed by the adolescent), the clinician is also inducing a self-reflection process from the beginning. In effect, the clinician tries to develop a process in which the adolescent does not have to feel submissive, and the adolescent can believe he or she has something worthwhile at stake. This approach fosters a sense of autonomy within a collaborative, interactive relationship—something that is typically novel to these adolescents.

Despite these efforts by the therapist, some adolescents may resist fully participating in the completion of the evaluation. This resistance confirms that the therapist cannot produce miracles and that the adolescent can be told, from the therapist's perspective, "Maybe you're not ready for this kind of work or therapy. The battle you want to win and your need to triumph may be the issue. It closes you off to others and them to you but also prevents you from learning about your self and others. I must still go ahead and discuss with your parents next steps they may want to consider."

The clinician communicates to the adolescent that the meeting that will be held with his or her parents will provide feedback about the clinician's recommendations based on the information that has been obtained. It should also be noted that even though therapy is not likely to proceed, planning will still occur and the adolescent's presence to listen to and engage in this discussion is welcomed and should be of interest to him or her. If the adolescent attends, the clinician can offer his or her perception, albeit incomplete, of the defensive dyad that is operating against the adolescent's true and full involvement. For someone like Anna, had she not eventually attended additional individual meetings that allowed for further elaboration and understanding of her interpersonal and identity problems, the feedback discussion based on the one meeting (prolonged individual and joint) she attended would have reflected the conflictual attachment issues that she had revealed that prevented her from experiencing true intimacy with parents or a romantic partner. The feedback discussion also would have shown how she undermined her attempts at this intimacy, which then raised the threats and fear of abandonment, and how she then turned the tables by making herself the inaccessible one and leaving her parents feeling anxious and abandoned. As a result, both she and her mother would feel anxious, angry, and helpless even though Anna was exercising omnipotent control. This shared negative emotion seemed to be the form of closeness they allowed themselves. For Anna, this interactive pattern allowed her to defend against revealing or even experiencing an unresolved or empty part of herself. Techniques we describe with some younger adolescents, such those used for addressing their refusal to talk, are applicable in the assessment phase as well.

For the therapist, it is important to be aware of possible projection by the adolescent and the parents and ensuing countertransference that can occur. Therapists should not be driven by feelings of helplessness or a sense of desperation to hold on to the patient because they have been made to feel frightened about the adolescent's well-being. The imagery of the adolescent's winning can still be utilized by pointing out that this victory does not stop the therapist from thinking, from trying to understand and be useful to the adolescent and family, and from expressing the hope that perhaps in the future the adolescent will be able to consider other points of view besides the one that has him or her trapped. The parents can be informed that the therapist does not feel there is more that he or she can do and that the therapist is wary that further pursuit of the adolescent, which can take on the quality of pleading, might just reinforce the adolescent's need to win. The parents can be helped to work out a plan/contract that expresses their needs and goals while also considering the needs of their child. This plan/contract can include their decisions and expectations about living arrangements, support for their child, school or work participation, and so forth and a clear indication of their next set of actions if their child does not fulfill such age-appropriate expectations. It may be useful for these very resistant adolescents and their families to see a different mental health worker to explore whether other pathways could be of value.

# Components of the Evaluation Process

The evaluation process may include a variety of procedures, although we will devote most of our attention to the clinical interviewing procedures used by TFP practitioners when examining features of personality organization. Taken together, these procedures allow the clinician to form a diagnostic impression that captures the distinguishing features of the adolescent and also develop a conclusion about the adolescent's level of personality organization, providing an impression of the severity of his or her problems. This is the information, to be described below, that informs the clinician's treatment recommendations.

Briefly, the assessment examines several components that are often part of a standard evaluation procedure with adolescents and that are relevant for understanding their current functioning. In addition, the TFP-A model provides an assessment of personality organization utilizing procedures that are unique to this goal. These multiple components include the following:

1. Identifying and examining the adolescent's symptomatology and behaviors that prompted the evaluation, including an overview of general functioning (e.g., mood, thinking, growth, health) as well as the adolescent's subjective experience of his or her anxiety, mood, and interpersonal relationships. The clinician then determines from this typical process how these findings conform to relevant nosology (e.g., DSM-5, ICD-10).
2. Functioning at school and/or work.
3. A thorough developmental history to identify the developmental phase of the onset of particular problems; long-term trends in the adolescent's functioning; family history of mood, anxiety, thought, and neurological disorders; the adolescent's medical history; and previous psychotherapy or pharmacological trials and the adolescent's responsiveness to these interventions. Contact with previous therapists, with parent and adolescent permission, is typically pursued. These inquiries are informed by a knowledge of risk factors for PD, especially BPD, in the life history of the adolescent and may include aspects of temperament (e.g., soothability, fearfulness, reaction to novelty, emotional control), history of trauma (e.g., sexual and physical abuse, medical trauma), neglect, loss (e.g., death of an important other), and the nature of the adolescent's attachment with caregivers (e.g., secure, disorganized).
4. Support systems, including relevant features of the parents' current level of functioning (e.g., employment, health, psychopathology, marital rela-

| **TABLE 4–1.** | **Core features of borderline personality disorder in adolescents** |
| --- | --- |

Significant abandonment fears

Unstable relationships that alternate between idealization and devaluation

Identity disturbance

Impulsivity that can be self-destructive

Recurrent suicidal behavior

Affective instability

Intense anger or difficulty controlling anger

Transient, stress-related paranoid orientation

Severe dissociative symptoms

Chronic feelings of emptiness

*Source.*    American Psychiatric Association 2013.

tionship) and parenting styles and the nature of their interaction with the patient and their other children.

5. Functioning with peers and with other social relations.
6. Observable behaviors and areas of dysfunction characteristic of BPD as described in DSM-5 (American Psychiatric Association 2013), which include both internal experiences and overt behaviors such as significant abandonment fears; unstable relationships that can alternate between idealization and devaluation; identity disturbance; impulsivity that could occur in ways that are self-destructive; recurrent suicidal behavior; affective instability; chronic feelings of emptiness; inappropriate intense anger or difficulty controlling anger; and transient, stress-related paranoid orientation or severe dissociative symptoms. Table 4–1 lists core features of BPD in adolescents.
7. The adolescent's level of personality organization. This is inferred by the clinician from his or her examination of underlying psychological structures while utilizing the Structural Interview (SI; Kernberg 1984) (see section "Assessment of Structure and Clinical Diagnostic Interviewing"), semi-structured interviewing (e.g., Structured Interview of Personality Organization—Revised [STIPO-R; Stern et al. 2018]), and the moment-to-moment interactions with the adolescent. The components of personality organization include identity status (diffusion/identity crisis), defensive operations, level of reality testing, aggressivity/sexuality, and moral development. The findings from the study of the adolescent's per-

sonality organization, informed by the severity of the problems in the development of these components, allow the therapist to draw conclusions about the level of borderline personality organization (BPO) and subsequent treatment recommendations.

# Standard Evaluation Procedures

The clinician can draw on semi-structured interviews and behavioral checklists so that information relevant to items 1–5 presented in the previous section can be obtained in a comprehensive and systematic fashion.

## Interview Format

While each clinician has his or her own personal approach to the evaluation process, a knowledge of the content and style described in standard semistructured interviews can be a helpful guide for areas to explore and possible approaches to inquiry. The Schedule for Affective Disorders and Schizophrenia for School-Age Children [K-SADS; Kaufman et al. 1997]) for example, while often used in research studies, provides the clinician with an awareness of the range of features that can and often should be inquired about and can serve as a "how to" guide that can be adapted to one's own personal style and needs.

## Checklist Format

Many checklists are available for clinical use and focus on different features of child and adolescent functioning, including mood (e.g., Beck Youth Inventories; Beck et al. 2005), attention (Conners 2008), and executive functioning (Barkley 2012). These checklists cover maladaptive traits and behaviors and can be administered efficiently, take relatively little of the respondent's time, cover a broad base of functioning, and allow for a comparison with normative expectations for the respondent's age. Checklists typically come in self, parent, and teacher formats, thereby providing information from multiple sources across different settings and perspectives. Therefore, the clinician can get a sense of whether there is a significant disparity between how the adolescent sees herself and how she is seen by others, whether she minimizes her observable problems, or whether the adults minimize or are unaware of the adolescent's internal problem (e.g., depressed mood) (Weiner 1983).

The ASEBA Child Behavior Checklist (CBCL; Achenbach 2006) is useful to consider. It has been fruitfully used in research with children and adolescents for decades and continues to receive prominent use. The CBCL offers self, parent, and teacher versions, and a young adult form is also available. The more than 100 items, when subjected to factor analysis, condense to eight factors and two superordinate factors, Internalizing and Externalizing. For those interested in ongoing research, the Internalizing and Externalizing dimensions are receiving increasing scrutiny (Sharp 2016; Sharp and Wall 2018), as is work examining factor group profiles (e.g., dysregulation profile—anxiety/depression, aggression, attention) and developmental patterns and outcomes (De Clercq et al. 2014). The CBCL can be informative to the clinician in several ways. Symptoms such as anxiety, depression, rule breaking, aggression, emotional instability, and avoidant cognitive strategies, which are associated with adolescent identity status (Crocetti et al. 2017), show considerable overlap with CBCL factors, and when the adolescent's responses are examined in a manner that goes beyond a simple factor score—when the meaning of a behavior is considered—alternative perspectives are possible. For example, Paulina Kernberg and colleagues (2000) pointed out that items from the CBCL such as "complains of loneliness; cruelty to others; deliberately harms self or attempts suicide; impulsive; sudden changes in mood; complains that no one loves him/her" are qualities seen in adolescents diagnosed with BPD. Therefore, CBCL results can go beyond meaningful factor scores and alert the clinician to PD features in the youngster who is being evaluated. It is particularly interesting that the CBCL items highlighted by Kernberg and colleagues load on both Internalizing and Externalizing factors. That these items are broadly distributed and not restricted to either Internalizing or Externalizing disorders appears consistent with recent factor analytic studies that show that BPD items may not constitute a single specific factor but are best seen as part of a general factor of psychopathology ("p" factor) that some also consider to be indicative of severity of pathology (Belsky et al. 2012; Sharp et al. 2015).

# Severity of Personality Pathology in the TFP-A Model

As discussed in Chapters 2 and 3, TFP ascribes an underlying structure to personality that reflects the individual's level of identity integration—the greater the degree of identity integration, the more the individual's personality approaches normal levels of functioning; the lower the level of integration, the more likely it is that the individual's personality organization is more pathological and associated with recognizable PD categories.

The TFP model utilizes traditional descriptive PD categories (e.g., those in DSM-5 Section II) while also recognizing the dimensional nature to psychopathology, and the model captures these two features with the concept of borderline level of personality organization (Caligor et al. 2018). The BPO dimension in adulthood ranges in severity from high, through mid-, to low levels. The neurotic personality organization (NPO) lies outside the boundary of BPO. We also adopt this configuration for describing differences among individual adolescents with regard to PD diagnostic categories and severity of impairment. As pathology gets more severe, individuals show decreased reflective capacity, empathy, and role taking, and increased splitting defenses; on interview they provide superficial, vague descriptions of self and other, perhaps just a few adjectives with "no meat on the bones." In effect, they have a superficial representation of others and cannot realize what the interviewer would need to know in order to have a well-rounded view of the individual they are describing. We will refer at times to individuals with NPO because they provide a useful frame of reference for understanding the range of BPO functioning.

Therefore, the BPO model is useful because it offers clinically informative descriptors as well as a severity dimension that may be useful for comparisons and judgments of change. The expectation is that BPO level is related to prognosis and change as the adolescent develops (i.e., those at a higher BPO level are generally expected to do better in these areas than those at lower BPO levels). In general, the more problematic the underlying structural organization, the greater the expectation of a more difficult treatment path and outcome, marked by less mature defenses, greater countertransference, more obvious expressions of transference, less control of affect and behavior, and therefore greater threats to the treatment contract.

Severity judgments impact several phases of the TFP-A treatment. Separate from the adolescent's underlying level of structural organization, contract formation will be affected by clinical judgments about the severity of some of the initial presenting problems. For example, is the adolescent currently using illicit drugs or alcohol, or does she have an eating disorder that is at a level that can be dealt with as part of the TFP-A treatment, or should she first go to a specialized program to get this problem under control and then begin TFP-A? Similarly, if there is self-injurious behavior, its severity will dictate the type of structure incorporated into the contract. To ensure familial support of the treatment, the assessment will determine if additional family interventions are needed.

With regard to the individual psychotherapy, clinicians can identify DSM-5 PD categories in adolescents, including borderline, narcissistic, avoidant, schizoid, and antisocial. Each of these individual PDs can range in severity, as conceptualized in the BPO model. For example, some adolescents with significant narcissistic features can include those with a low level of BPO, meaning there is considerable identity diffusion and elements of a pathological grandiose self (Diamond et al. 2011), whereas other adolescents with narcissistic personality qualities can be organized at a higher level of BPO. The following brief vignettes illustrate narcissistic PD in adolescents that fall at different levels of severity on the BPO dimension. These cases will then be referred to as we proceed to describe how features of BPD may be manifested at different BPO levels.

# Illustrations of Narcissistic PD at Different Levels of Borderline Personality Organization

**High BPO:** This 16-year-old had been marginally responsive when treated with psychotherapy and medication for his depression and anxiety. He was unengaged with peers and schoolwork, and therapists, school personnel, and parents were concerned that he was fragile and possibly psychotic and that it would be detrimental if more was demanded of him. An evaluation that eventually recognized and confronted his manipulativeness and hostility that was masked by his passivity fostered self-awareness of his anger. He then became more in touch with and expressive about his narcissistic concerns—that if he allowed himself aspirations but failed, it would bring more shame on him and his family; and that he was embarrassed about his home, which was disheveled because of his parents' inadequacies. Therefore, he did not make friends and so did not have to bring friends home. He articulated wishes to be able to have friends and go out with girls but felt he might have to wait to do this until he went to college and was away from home and disentangled from the reputation he had at school. Although he still had significant anxiety and problems to confront, he appeared much healthier than originally thought and was not psychotic.

**Mid-BPO:** This 16-year-old was brought for an evaluation because of aggression toward peers and disrespect toward teachers—actions that were unusual in his private school. His mother felt she was "walking on eggshells" in his presence. In evaluation, he complained that many of his teachers were "idiots," that he was more knowledgable than many of them, and that he and his group of friends were smarter than the others in his grade. The defense of splitting was often expressed but not in severe forms. His devaluation of others, self-aggrandizement, and hostility were soon expressed in the transference. He displayed the defense of omnipotent control by his refusal to talk or respond to questions. The clinician attempted to discuss this non-responsiveness with him, but after one particular inquiry this adolescent commented, "What book did you get that from? Notice I didn't say books because it's in all of them!" The implication was that he had read all the relevant texts and was just checking on the one the clinician had read! Thus, the devaluation was coupled with grandiosity and hostility. The evaluation also indicated that while he was verbally aggressive and hostile to his mother, he also felt warmth and enjoyed certain activities with her but was restrained in expressing positive affect. He typically avoided his father (parents were divorced) because he could not tolerate being in the presence of the father's expression of anxiety, but there were certain activities they could enjoy together (e.g., going to a sporting event).

**Low BPO:** This 15-year-old had few acquaintances and no close friends. He tended to avoid closeness with parents and those siblings that were closest in age to him. He did not ask for things from parents (their complaint) but complained they did not give him anything and were nonresponsive (his complaint), a pattern that guaranteed their angry distance from one another, although the adolescent knew his parents loved him and were "good people." He refused to keep up with schoolwork, prepare for exams, or willingly help out at home. He constantly portrayed himself as the victim in all dyads and expressed a paranoid quality about most relations, including the belief that classmates were jealous of him. Splitting defense was prominent and associated with moments of poorer judgments of reality. He could not allow closeness, mutual nurturance, and dependency. His omnipotent control was expressed more pervasively and intensely than was seen with the patient with mid-BPO, as were his expressions of rage (e.g., punching a hole in a wall at home). He painfully experienced intense emptiness, which he distinguished from depressed mood. He was not responsive to antidepressants or stimulants, or to small doses of atypical antipsychotic medication. The narcissistic elements were expressed via his complaints of classmates' ignorance or superficiality and teachers inadequacies. For example, on one exam, rather than writing an analysis of the book that was read, he wrote a critique of how the teacher should have taught the material and was surprised that the teacher and the school administrators reacted angrily rather than being grateful for his help. As the treatment proceeded, he expressed his belief that unless one was the best in the world at something, "why bother?"

For purposes of comparison, the description of a high school student with NPO is also presented below. He requested psychotherapy because he was shy and anxious and wanted to try to modify these features before he went off to college. He, like others with NPO, may be more likely than those who fall on the BPO dimension to initiate the referral because they have the tendency to reflect on their problem and find it ego dystonic, can envision a more desirable alternative, and, though they may feel anxious and "weird" about entering treatment, are less likely to feel frightened about forming a relationship with the therapist. Their referral often derives from a joint decision between parent and adolescent.

# Illustration of Adolescent With NPO

This 17-year-old was midway through his final year of high school when he first came for psychotherapy. He was a bright and successful student who was planning to go to college the next year. He offered a clear presentation of his problem and of himself. He said his reason for pursuing psychotherapy was that he was extremely anxious, always had been (as was his father), and was concerned that his shyness and anxiety would interfere with his success and enjoyment at college. He thought his shyness had been having that effect in high school. For example, he had an editorial role on a school publication but did not feel comfortable or know how to confront students who ignored his editorial directions; he had heterosexual interests but had not asked any girl out, nor could he seem to imagine how to approach his wish to have a date and attend his senior prom. He was able to successfully attend overnight summer camps, so he did not appear to have significant separation anxiety. His shyness was confronted— how did he reconcile his image that he was shy with the fact that he joined the publication staff and pursued an editorial position? This led to a reconceptualization of how he saw himself, with the realization that his conflict was over being aggressive in a variety of situations, which typically prevented him from taking the initiative to act on his wish. He was pleasant to be with, respectful toward the therapist, and motivated to try new ideas. For example, after he was accepted at a college, he asked if he should join a gathering of other new students that was being held in his area. Thus, he was willing to seek advice and be dependent in the service of growth.

# Assessment of Structure and Clinical Diagnostic Interviewing

Table 4–2 shows five basic components about which the clinician makes a dimensional assessment in order to determine the adolescent's BPO level. By obtaining a sense of the severity of the problem in each area, the clinician can formulate a diagnostic impression and determine the possible BPO level for that individual that will guide feedback to the patient, indicate an approach to treatment, and contribute to expectations about prognosis. In this section we describe how these five features appeared along the BPO spectrum in the three teenagers presented earlier in this chapter. We then demonstrate how the SI (Kernberg 1984; Yeomans et al. 2015) and the Personality Assessment Inventory (PAI; Selzer et al. 1987) can be deployed to examine these features that contribute to the picture of an individual's personality as understood by the TFP model.

## Determination of BPO Status

A determination of the adolescent's identity status as a reflection of his or her level of structural organization is a fundamental goal of the TFP-A assessment process. Because adolescence is conceptualized as a developmental phase in which the establishment of behavioral independence and a sense of autonomy is expected to occur when processes that propel separation-individuation are active, one wonders what a "healthy" sense of self would look like amid such profound transformations that are fundamental to an individual's self representation? It must be acknowledged that concepts such as "stable" or "well integrated" may seem incongruous for describing an adolescent's identity status during a period in which these very processes are expected to be changing. Clearly, the clinician should not make comparisons with adult models or consider how far the adolescent is from an adult norm. Instead, while still within the context of unfolding developmental processes, the clinician will judge how integrated or confusing and chaotic the adolescent's response is, whether it makes sense, and whether there are contradictions and inconsistencies—in effect, how well organized and integrated is the adolescent's description about himself or herself and others as compared with what is offered by better-functioning adolescents of the same developmental level? What does the process and organization of the

| TABLE 4-2. | Fundamental component processes of borderline personality organization status determination |
|---|---|

Identity formation

Object relations

Defenses

Aggression—expression and management

Moral functioning

response indicate about this adolescent's inner life, his or her construction of self and others, and defenses independent of how dramatic or mundane the content of his or her response?

Adolescence may cover a relatively brief period, but it represents almost half of the individual's lifetime, and so it is reasonable to formulate different expectations for early and late adolescence because there are different contributors to development at these milestone points. Younger adolescents are experiencing rapid change: biologically based changes produce transformations in a physical self, and the body in which they live is changing; it feels different to them, and they are experienced as different and changing by others. Furthermore, peers are changing at different rates, providing the "opportunity" for constant comparison and self-judgment. Comments from others—such as "You're getting so big; I can hardly recognize you," "What are you going to do now that you're growing up?" "Do you have a boyfriend/girlfriend yet?"—reflect how the world has begun to see them as changing and is reacting to them differently, including having changing expectations for them. Erikson (1968) noted the importance of society's recognition and acceptance of the changes adolescents are experiencing and of the way in which they present their self to the world. Older adolescents have now experienced many of these changes, have integrated them into a sense of self in some way, and are trying to move on to testing this new but still changing self in different situations as a way of discovering more about who they are. Do they discover a quality of constancy across all these changes and transitions—a sense of continuity, a feeling of sameness that "this is me, who I am" (not "who am I?")?

The evaluative process seeks to examine how this quality is developing in the adolescent. In addition, the cognitive changes of adolescence allow for a more abstract orientation that not only permits a conceptualization of the world as it is but also allows for a recognition of how it might be or could have been—in these "other worlds," if I had had other parents, attributes, and so forth. "Could I change my current situation, and, if so, to what?" So, while we might try to determine if the adult has a stable experience of himself or herself (Caligor et al. 2018), with adolescents we try to determine whether they have a consistent sense of self for this period of their life and whether they can experience and recognize continuity of self amid the change—that "I am still the me I have known amid the change in my external and internal appearance and experience (my voice, the hair on my body, my sexuality, feelings toward others)." Is the future that they imagine one that is appealing or alarming? These issues may be magnified for those adolescents who mature much more quickly or slowly than the norm. For example, one very rapidly developing teenage male, who grew tall and developed secondary sexual characteristics very quickly and could grow a beard before many classmates had any need to shave, viewed himself as a "monster," thought others did as well, and could not imagine that other boys might be jealous of his growth or that some girls might consider him to be mature and attractive. All of these concepts are pursued when the adolescent is asked, "Tell me what brings you here. What is your understanding of why we are meeting? Tell me about yourself."

## Severity and Identity Status

When using terms such as "high functioning" and "low functioning," unless otherwise indicated, we are referring to the adolescent's level of structural organization and not to concepts such as cognitive or intellectual functioning. Responses that reflect higher-level borderline organization display healthier object relations, less pervasive or intense aggression, and more age-appropriate moral functioning, suggesting a context of less identity diffusion.

Those at a lower level of personality organization display more severe identity diffusion, as reflected in their more pervasive use of defenses such as splitting, projective identification, omnipotent control, and devaluation of others, including the therapist; a stronger paranoid orientation; and a quality to their object representations that reflects their compromised ability to establish good interpersonal relations and greater difficulty interpreting social cues and being empathic, along with more significant aggression and possible dissociative experiences. Their object relations and defenses can result in more labile emotional expression than is observed at the neurotic level or higher borderline level because of the shifting levels of ego functioning that result. This observation is consistent with the view that emotional dysregulation is one of the core factors in the development of a PD (Putnam and Silk 2005). Feelings of emptiness, dysphoria, and often a lack of pleasure or nonresponsiveness to praise or rewards are also present in adolescents at lower levels of BPO.

Regarding the evaluation of identity status, higher-functioning adolescents can often describe themselves in a fairly comprehensive manner, and the clinician does not have to work hard to obtain descriptions that typically offer a nonfragmented, realistic, understandable picture of who they are and what their concerns are. For example, the adolescent with NPO described earlier in this chapter readily spoke about his anxiety, his reasons for entering therapy, and his goals. He clearly and easily described his life, the range of his activities, and how he saw himself in different settings. The adolescent with high BPO level at first could not. He was avoidant and extremely passive and used these qualities in a manipulative, controlling manner. However, he showed a remarkably different reaction after these qualities were confronted. Rather than regressing or avoiding this intervention, he was able to move on to demonstrate a somewhat healthier internal structure by providing a more comprehensive, and therefore more integrated and adaptive, picture of himself in which he described his self-consciousness, his concerns about shame, how he wished things were, and his clearer understanding of the relationship between his parents' behaviors and his own. In effect, this adolescent's organization was at a higher level than initially expected, and he could reveal his functioning at this level in a more structured situation in which he felt safe, following the utilization of the techniques of clarification and confrontation. The use of these two techniques is not restricted to therapy proper, and their impact will greatly depend on the adolescent's structural level.

Adolescents at lower levels of BPO provide more vague descriptions of self and other that are experienced by the clinician as fragmented. It is as if one were looking at a mosaic that has some tiles but is missing many others, so that the viewer has to work hard to create or imagine a full image. Similarly, interviewing these youngsters requires a lot of thought and action from the clinician. As seen with the mid-BPO adolescent earlier, the clinician had to do a great deal of work just to get him to talk, and with both the mid- and low-BPO adolescents, the clinician had to provide constant structure and support to try to draw from them more pieces for the mosaic and to determine how unintegrated their identity might be. The mid-BPO adolescent in our example was not talkative except when he offered his hostile devaluation of the clinician; the low-BPO adolescent was more talkative but restricted himself to angry diatribes about family, teachers, and peers and struggled to offer a broader picture of himself. In effect, both of these youngsters showed a more rigid approach to interacting with the clinician and offered a narrower picture of themselves. The low-BPO adolescent also provided a unidirectional picture of causality: he was the constant victim. The high-BPO youngster's default response was "I don't know" until he altered his replies following confrontation of his manipulative lying, showing some degree of flexibility; the low-BPO adolescent's default position was an angry characterization of his victimizers and his belief that everything was their fault. The rigidity with which he applied this response style indicated his deficit in mentalizing and an inability to consider how others were perceiving his reactions to them.

It should be noted that the mid- and low-BPO adolescents in these examples were extremely intelligent, well read, and knowledgable about many subjects (despite their variable or constant refusal to do schoolwork), yet their responses could at times be fragmented. It can be tempting for the clinician to believe he or she knows what patients mean and unwittingly "clean up" their replies. It may be especially so with such intelligent adolescents and, conversely, could be less so with others who are less articulate or intelligent. A variation on this theme was seen with another intelligent 16-year-old male who demonstrated how one's presentation can change across the session and thereby provide a clarifying picture of the patient's identity status. This adolescent told about his decision to reenter psychotherapy to a new, prospective therapist. He sounded assured and mature in his decision making and seemed to display good self-awareness even in describing his mediocre school performance characterized by his holding himself back in tackling his assignments. As he proceeded he revealed that he very frequently lied and used marijuana twice daily but had (proudly) given it up (but later in the discussion indicated that was just 3 weeks previous), and the more he spoke, the more striking became the vagueness of his comments. His self-portrayal demonstrates that the organization of self is also independent of the adolescent's language skill, and, therefore, an expressive language disorder means not that the adolescent will necessarily present as disorganized or chaotic nor that being articulate will automatically mask identity diffusion and an internal emptiness. An awareness of these tendencies helps prevent the clinician from overlooking the disorganization or fragmentation associated with BPO status.

Part of identity assessment will include an examination of goals. Young children may often be asked, "What do you want to be when you grow up?" Today, this question for many adolescents is fraught with anxiety because of the pressure they feel to establish a career/job path or qualify for higher education at the school of their choice. An evaluation of adolescents' capacity to pursue goals will include a judgment of how realistic their choices are: Are their choices consistent with their abilities? Will their choice provide satisfaction (as opposed to being a feature of identity foreclosure done just to please others)? Do the goals make sense for their developmental level (i.e., do they offer only long-term unrealistic or grandiose goals, or can they also say, for example, "I want to be a counselor at this camp this summer")? Do they take appropriate initiative to achieve the goal, or do they depend too much on others for help? Can they carry out their part even if helped? In effect, can they identify short- and long-term goals that are realistic, and can they conceive of how to pursue them? These are features that can be distinguished from those in adolescents who cannot imagine a goal or how to make it happen (even how to ask for help with homework or with seeking a part-time job) and reflect Erikson's description of time and work diffusion as components of identity diffusion. These are the individuals who may be described as "poor planners," but labeling them as such may miss the essence of the issue here, which involves more of a sense that they "have all the time in the world" or "never have enough time to get it done" and also have grandiose or dismaying expectations of themselves in their effort, both of which are unrealistic.

The clinician may try to distinguish between the role of anxiety derived from a parenting style that made few demands or had low expectations and fostered dependency and one that promoted more insecure attachment patterns that engendered avoidant techniques and a poor sense of how to navigate the world. Those with more severe pathology will have greater difficulty formulating or establishing goals and feeling comfort and excitement in pursuing them, but may display what seems like task- and situation-appropriate anxiety. At its core for some of these late adolescents/ young adults is a dread of adulthood expressed and manifested in a variety of ways.

## Severity and Object Relations

The impact of the severity of pathology on representation of others is similar to its impact on self representation. At lower levels of BPO the adolescent's description of others can often be vague, perhaps just the listing of a few adjectives with "no meat on the bones." Furthermore, these adolescents typically do not have an appreciation for the listener's need to know more in order to have a true image of the other person they are supposed to be describing. Because of their superficial representation of others, they often exhibit a void, an absence of understanding of why the clinician is asking for more and a limited awareness of what could be offered to provide a more well-rounded picture of another person. It is as if they do not have a sense of what else is needed in the "mosaic" to make it visible and knowable to the other, again demonstrating another feature of their poor mentalization. Some adolescents, especially younger ones, may be helped by a kind of "scaffolding" technique that gives them greater distance from the question. For example, if they struggle with "tell me about yourself," they might be told, "Suppose someone asked a friend of yours to tell them about you; how do you think they would describe you?" or "What should they know about you so that they get a good sense of who you really are and what you are like?"

The inquiry also seeks to know if the adolescent can get close to others— can he or she sustain a relationship and pursue mutuality rather than be exploitative? Mastering and internalizing these qualities requires a degree of empathy, the ability to care for others and to be able to depend on and be depended on. Giving and receiving gifts, for adults as well as adolescents, can be an excellent indicator of conflicts about dependency and nurturance. The adolescent with low BPO described earlier, while often complaining how deprived and neglected he was, hated to receive gifts and refused to make his wishes known. He felt that if one received something, there was an automatic obligation to reciprocate, and that raised the dilemma that what he gave back might not be liked by the recipient. It was as if he could not imagine that other persons would want to give him something merely because they cared for him or that they would appreciate what he gave to them merely because he thought of them and wanted to please them with his gift. Instead, his wariness with regard to features of mutuality reflected a paranoid orientation.

In the clinical examples earlier in this chapter, the high-BPO patient was socially withdrawn and anxious about relationships and had few friends but was able to present his sense of the friendships he longed for, with male friends as well as girlfriends. He was able to give a somewhat nuanced view of his parents. The low-BPO patient provided a restricted, unidimensional representation of others. His brother was described as a selfish, greedy "pain" who gets whatever he wants; classmates were described as arrogant and entitled. His brother was seen as not smart and got away with it and received parental support and understanding for his deficiencies; classmates were not really knowledgeable or as smart as they thought; teachers were inept and unfair; parents were demanding only of him and not of his siblings; he got nothing and his siblings got everything. Thus, this cast of characters may have different names and roles but are essentially presented as having little differentiation among them—he is the deprived, under-appreciated, shamed victim, and they are all selfish and demanding, yet reap rewards, and are unempathic, justifying his enraged, aggressive stance toward the world. The mid-BPO adolescent was able to have friends, his "posse," who were like him in being smarter than the others. He did not offer much else in his portrayal of them beyond their superiority over other classmates, thereby supporting his more grandiose self-portrayal. Unlike the low-BPO youngster, the mid-BPO adolescent offered a more well-rounded view of his parents. While he expressed his annoyance and disappointment in each of them, he also noted positive qualities that drew him to engage in certain activities with each parent.

The NPO adolescent described earlier did not have many friends that he spent much time with, but his higher level of structural organization was evident in his full description of classmates he shared assignments with and his depiction of a girl he hoped to ask out. It was clear to the interviewer what this girl was like and why she appealed to him. Perhaps reflective of his level of dependency and anxiety level, his description of his parents was narrow and emphasized their need-fulfilling roles. In contrast to the mid- and low-BPO adolescents, his aggression was contained, both behaviorally and expressively, and as might have been expected, the rigid inhibition associated with his conflict over expressing aggression/assertiveness contributed to his anxiety and the pursuit of psychotherapy.

## Severity and Defenses

Paulina Kernberg (1994) provided a list of 31 defense mechanisms used by children and adolescents that ranged from normal through neurotic, borderline, and psychotic levels. These defense mechanisms constitute the child's and adolescent's familiar ways of coping with or adapting to their external stressors and internal conflicts. She cited a study by Jacobson et al. (1986), who reported that nonpatients utilized defenses such as altruism, suppression, and intellectualization, whereas adolescent psychiatric patients were more likely to resort to acting out, avoidance, displacement, projection, and turning against the self. Thus, the nonpatients utilized defenses that were classified at the normal level by Kernberg, while patients deployed defenses that were likely to be seen as neurotic or borderline and were consistent with the adolescent's level of ego development. These findings demonstrate that choice of defense mechanisms can be distinguished among groups of adolescents and that the defenses ultilized correlate with severity of pathology.

The developmental model of PDs presented in Chapter 2 described the defensive role that splitting plays under certain peak affect experiences. In the adolescent and adult, splitting-based defenses can be distinguished from repression-based defenses associated with higher-level BPO and NPO. The divisions in their self- and object-world made by the individual with BPD are quickly evident to the interviewer. Their black-white/good-bad descriptions draw the interviewer's attention to the contradictions in the patient's mental life. For example, our mid-level BPO adolescent immediately described the split between his "good/smart" friends and the "bad/inept" other students and teachers. The low-BPO adolescent made similar distinctions about others that were also captured in the object representations of the "good/victimized" self and the "bad/victimizing" teachers and parents. These adolescents also utilized splitting-based defenses (Caligor et al. 2018) such as omnipotent control, projective identification, and idealization/devaluation as experienced by the interviewer in the countertransference. The mid-BPO adolescent demonstrated the omnipotent control through his silence; the low-BPO adolescent did it through his rageful complaining that he described as his need to "vent." However, the venting controlled the conversation and was an attempt to avoid having to reflect on and answer the interviewer's inquiries. The mid-BPO adolescent's devaluation was expressed in a direct "put down" of the interviewer, an attempt to humiliate the interviewer with a comment that was simultaneously self-aggrandizing; the low-BPO patient typically maintained his superiority by showing how knowledgeable he was and by generally finding fault in the clinician's comments and interpretations. This adolescent always had to be the one who was correct. The high-BPO youngster showed omnipotent control and projective identification, which was experienced by his therapist and psychiatrist, leaving them fearful of pushing him toward further regressed behavior or breakdown. However, the confrontation by the evaluator resulted in a flexible movement away from this pattern, demonstrating greater health than was imagined.

Splitting defenses create the vague, superficial presentations that make these adolescents more difficult to follow. It is as if this defense keeps items in separate compartments, where they can be thought about and dealt with individually in isolation from other contradictory representations. But the clinician's use of confrontation does not accept this coping method, and the adolescent is now asked to reflect on the internal and external experiences, behaviors, and communications that created these constructions of his or her world that do not fit, that are inconsistent because this defense tries to keep these contradictions outside of awareness. The confrontation will make the adolescent uncomfortable because the adolescent's familiar but unconscious adaptation is now shown not to be working and he or she must reflect and search for another approach to coping.

Simultaneously, some of these adolescents may feel frustrated by their ineffective attempts to explain themselves and satisfy the clinician's questions, provoking an angry reaction in them because they may feel the other is attempting to make them look foolish. The vagueness that results from splitting is to be distinguished from the withholding and hostile resistance some adolescents may show, which may be reflected in the countertransference as feeling provoked or controlled rather than confused or uncertain. Younger adolescents may also experience higher levels of egocentrism, which Elkind (1967) noted can include the creation of a "collective audience," the belief of adolescents that others are thinking about what they are thinking about (typically themselves). Perhaps this contributes to some adolescents believing that the clinician will automatically, almost magically, understand them and as a result not appreciating the need to be explicit in order to be understood.

Confrontation should not be seen as an angry or judgmental challenge or a criticism of adolescents' response. It is, in effect, reflecting back to these patients things they said or did but which they were trying to keep separate, outside of simultaneous awareness. Thus, the clinician is not making an inference but is asking these adolescents to look at what came from them, what they generated; by doing this, the clinician is moving these adolescents toward self-reflection by first providing them with a reflection of themselves.

These splitting defenses can be distinguished from repression-based defenses that are more likely to be seen in individuals with NPO. Our NPO adolescent was seen to use these repression-based defenses to keep himself unaware of the conflicts he felt about aggressive, assertive/competitive, and hostile urges. The high-BPO adolescent also used these defenses, and they led to his anxiety, avoidance, and passivity and his restricted impulse expression. Both the low- and high-BPO individuals were sensitive and experienced significant shame. The high-BPO adolescent could eventually talk about it and lead the interviewer to these themes as he became more reflective following the use of clarification and confrontation, whereas the low-BPO adolescent would become more enraged in order to block the experience and expression of these feelings.

## Severity and Aggression

Adolescence can be seen as a time both to develop and to modulate the expression of aggression. Aggression is expressed in different forms with different functions and differing underlying neurobiological substrates (e.g., play fighting, dominance, aspects of the "seeking" system, as well as being intertwined with sexuality) (Panksepp and Biven 2012). Adolescents, male and female, will need to further develop and refine their expression of aggression so that they can express anger and rage in an appropriate manner when this feeling is justifiable; engage in competition on the sports field, in the classroom, and in relationships; and combine aggression with tenderness as they move toward sexually intimate relationships.

A great deal about the adolescent's prior and current expressions of aggression will be learned when the clinician asks the adolescent to provide his or her understanding of the reason for this meeting. The reply often includes a description of aggression or hostile behaviors toward others, self-harming or dangerous behaviors, and displays of hostile speech with the interviewer. However, patients may deny or hide any aggressive or violent history, so the interviewer needs to ask about the diverse ways in which aggression can be expressed because it is an important contributor to diagnostic thinking and treatment planning. Thus, inquiry should be made about suicidality, self-cutting, or other acts that cause bodily pain or harm; eating problems such as bingeing and purging; dangerous or risky behaviors, such as unsafe sex or associating with peers who get into trouble; amount of alcohol and drug use; and direct expressions of aggression toward others, including loss of temper and overt aggression (assault/bullying). Expressions of aggression that occur on an internal level, such as extreme feelings of envy and thoughts of revenge, can also be asked about (Caligor et al. 2018).

The adolescents in the clinical examples in this chapter displayed different features of aggression consistent with their level of pathology. More severe personality pathology is associated with more inappropriate, intense, and pervasive expressions of aggression. The adolescent diagnosed with NPO experienced considerable conflict over the expression of aggression. A major contributor to his anxiety was his strong discomfort with his wish to be assertive—to tell others what to do as part of his role in a publication and to be more forceful when met by refusal, and to be more direct in asking a girl to go out with him. The high-BPO youngster also experienced conflict over the expression of aggression, but unlike the adolescent with NPO, he used even more severe defenses that prevented any expression of assertiveness and a denial of any wishes to pursue action. Thus, the impact was more pervasive for him.

Both the mid- and low-BPO adolescents overtly expressed aggression. They each refused to comply with others' expectations (e.g., regarding schoolwork) and overtly were hostile toward others, including parents and peers. Each was resistant and demeaning toward teachers but in different ways. The mid-BPO youngster appeared to restrict it to certain teachers whom he thought were unworthy of his respect, while the low-BPO adolescent showed a more pervasive disdain for others that was coupled with a broader refusal of compliance. The mid-BPO adolescent may have been more hostile toward a small group of peers, while the low-BPO youngster showed a more pervasive avoidance of others and extreme discomfort with being appropriately assertive toward male and female peers and therefore had no true friendships. Most apparent was the low-BPO adolescent's more pervasive and intense level of hostility. He was angry at most people most of the time, drove family members to avoid him because of this, and became so angry that he punched a hole in a wall at home. These examples indicate the value of careful investigation of this area of functioning because of its contribution to understanding the severity of an adolescent's personality pathology.

# Severity and Moral Functioning

Adolescence includes developmental changes in moral functioning that can be described according to different theoretical assumptions that include behaviors, features of conscience attributed to superego development, and moral judgments offered for moral behaviors (Weiner 2006). These components, when viewed integratively, can be informative when the clinician is evaluating an adolescent's moral functioning. For example, Caligor and colleagues (2018) point out that some individuals may base their moral actions on the fear of being caught, while other's actions or justifications imply a more internalized value system. These patterns are reminiscent of Kohlberg's developmental model of moral judgments in young people (Kohlberg and Kramer 1969). On the basis of individuals' responses to moral dilemmas that did not have a "right" or "wrong" answer, Kohlberg classified their moral judgments into three levels that described a transition from developmentally less mature (i.e., "preconventional") judgments that emphasized what was in one's own best interest, with little awareness of others' needs (e.g., "I could get into trouble if I did X; I should do X because it would satisfy my basic need of…"), to a developmental level that reflected accepted convention (e.g., "I should do/not do X because then people would think I'm a good/bad person"), to a highly principled level (e.g., "I might get into trouble for doing X, but doing X reflects universal human principles that transcend the moment, such as saving a life"). Transitions across these three levels occur with development. Similarly, conscience development (Jacobson 1964) can include a transition toward greater internalization from a position of identification such that the older adolescent has the potential to experience useful guilt and other emotions that result neither in ignoring conventions nor in harsh and restrictive self-criticism. The implication is that a developmental perspective provides a needed framework when the clinician is evaluating an adolescent's moral functioning.

Our NPO adolescent's conscience restricted his impulse expression by constraining his acting on age-appropriate sexual and aggressive impulses. However, because his object relations were well integrated, he could imagine pursuing his romantic interests and sexual feelings with a specific girl whom he could describe in a manner that clearly represented who she was and why she appealed to him. This is contrasted with the low-BPO adolescent, who was physically mature and had strong sexual interests (indeed, he commented that "masturbation is probably the only normal thing I do") but could not let himself approach a girl. He acted very appropriately away from his school in school-sponsored events, and as a result, several girls appeared to show interest in him, but he did not follow up beyond making brief conversations with them at these events. So, while he would emphatically exclaim, "I want to get fucked!," he could not modulate his rage to be able to pursue a relationship and could not imagine anyone he thought appealing would find him interesting—they would only view him as a "hairy monster." Both of these young men can be contrasted with another who struggled over a moral dilemma. There was a girl who he knew was interested enough to want to be sexually involved with him, but he did not care for her, in part because he did not believe she was well regarded by his peers and so being with her was not prestigious. Thus, his struggle included two features: should he "hook up" with her and risk imagined ridicule for his choice, or should he "hook up" with someone he did not strongly like but who liked him and thereby "take advantage" of someone in a way that would violate his developing moral principles and which he would feel guilty about? This discussion illustrates how a complex issue such as sexuality involves considering how the adolescent's level of aggression, defensive organization, representation of self and other, and level of moral development can interact to determine his or her behavior.

In a more straightforward manner, the clinician can ask the adolescent whether he or she lies or steals, or has physically harmed another, especially when there are hints of that in the interview. These are also complex acts that may represent different levels of severity. For example, one adolescent boy described stealing sunglasses in a store during a class trip. He then gave the glasses to a girl in his group. It turned out that he did not do this to impress the girl or get her to like him. Instead, he said he disliked the store owner, whom he thought was rude to his classmate, so he stole the glasses just to demonstrate that he could do this and then felt superior to the owner because he believed he made the store owner look foolish. Here, narcissistic needs drove this antisocial act in a mid- to high-BPO youngster. This greatly contrasts with the behavior of a 17-year-old young man who despised his divorced parents, frequently lied, and attempted to truly deceive the interviewer, while portraying himself as the victim of an uncaring and ungiving father who was also described as nasty toward his beleaguered ex-wife. When the young man was confronted about his inconsistencies regarding his frequent marijuana use, it became clear he was also engaging in criminal activity by dealing drugs at his school. This significant antisocial action also served oedipal goals because he could maintain a belief that he was more financially successful than his struggling father. This level of antisocial behavior, as is the case with significant antisocial behavior in adults, suggests a poorer prognosis (Caligor et al. 2018). An attempt at TFP-A with an adolescent like this would require a carefully constructed contract, well-defined parental involvement, and the adolescent's motivation in pursuing treatment goals. In addition, because this adolescent, a minor, was involved in illegal activities that had the risk of personal harm and significant legal consequences, it would be necessary to explain to him the need to discuss this with his parents and involve them in a plan to ensure his safety.

# Additional Contributing Features to the Assessment Process

Table 4–2 listed the core components that guide clinicians' inquiries and contribute to their conclusions about the patient's BPO level. Our description of this evaluation process also alluded to other contributing elements, which we now address. Table 4–3 includes additional features that either present themselves or can be asked about during the assessment interviews and that contribute to the clinician's understanding of the adolescent and inform inferences about BPO level. Many of these contributors have been referred to previously in the course of describing various other elements. Here we will primarily focus on supportive relationships. Suffice it to say that content such as body image and topics related to sexuality are directly inquired about, often as a follow-up to something the adolescent has mentioned and when expansion or clarification are in order. The other items in Table 4–3 are typically inferred from the adolescent's responses to the interviewing process.

| TABLE 4–3. | Additional contributors to severity assessment |
|---|---|

Supportive relationships (family and peers—e.g., comfort with intimacy; enmeshment or distancing)

Narcissism

Integration of sexuality (in self and romantic relationships)

Reflective capacity (toward self and other)

Body image

Rigidity/inhibition vs. flexibility

Affect regulation

An evaluation of the adolescent's family, school functioning, and social world can help to determine if the personality pathology displayed by the adolescent could be reflective of poor differentiation from family pathology or a merging with and adoption of peer group features (Kernberg et al. 1992). If either of these is the case, a therapeutic goal would involve helping the adolescent recognize this situation, including the possibility that his or her best interests are served by separation from these destructive relationships, rather than the more expected goal of enhancing closeness between adolescent and family or peers.

# Parents

Here too, as with the evaluation of the adolescent himself or herself, a fundamental goal of the clinician is to assess the severity of pathology of the parents and the family unit, to have a sense of how the concept of personality organization applies to these contributors to the adolescent's life. This will inform how the clinician can best interact with the parents in order to enlist their support for the treatment and to determine how often it is necessary to meet with them and for what goals, as well as to ascertain whether additional interventions by other clinical services are needed (e.g., individual psychotherapy for the parent[s], family therapy). It may also be necessary to prepare the parents to support other interventions (e.g., management of alcohol or drug use, treatment of eating disorders) that may need to precede the initiation of TFP-A proper.

The evaluation of family functioning, including sibling relations, contributes to understanding the development of the adolescent's personality as well as determining the parents' or others' ability to participate in and support the adolescent's psychotherapy. Support would include the parents' ability and willingness to pay for the therapy and to ensure that their child has a way of getting to therapy regularly and on time. It is ideal to establish expectations and procedures during the contracting phase that foster the adolescent's ability to be in charge of transportation to and from psychotherapy sessions. This way, it is primarily the adolescent's resistance that will have to be dealt with as part of the therapy. It is much more difficult when a parent's resistance invades the therapy, because the clinician must deal with the parent as well as with the adolescent's possible conflicted feelings about the parent's acting out.

Therapy can be supported or undermined by the parent in subtle ways. For example, one mother of a 15-year-old boy would pick up her son after school and drive 45 minutes to get to each therapy session, yet, despite his repeated requests, she would not bring her "starving" son an after-school snack for the car ride, so he decided to "go on strike" and remain in the car rather than enter therapy. Her preferred mode was to buy the snack after they arrived so she could interrupt the session and give it to him. Her pattern reflected her stated wish that he improve and stop being aggressive and insulting toward her (therefore, she brought him to therapy), but she could not relinquish control and allow for his separation and true growth, so she undermined therapy, especially after he began to improve and show a positive reaction to his therapist. She attributed the problem to her busy schedule and her ADHD, which she asserted promoted disorganization and prevented her from effective planning that would have allowed her to get the snack. Her own PD played a larger role by promoting continued conflict with her son.

This mother's action is similar to research findings from studies of mothers diagnosed with BPD. These mothers have difficulty fostering autonomy and relatedness because of deficits in engaging with their teenage child and validating their opinions; they inhibit the development of autonomy by overpersonalizing disagreements, which reduces independent thought and behavior; and they deal with their fear of abandonment by keeping their child close, often via hostile interactions, and thereby undermine their child's development of relatedness and independence (Frankel-Waldheter et al. 2015). These types of interactions would also be expected to impair the healthy development of mentalization. Parents' general attitude about their child's movement toward separation and autonomy can often be explored by asking them whether they reacted with joy, or hesitancy and disappointment, when their child comfortably experienced a significant developmental milestone (e.g., entering high school).

In addition to hearing about the parents' fears of and for their child, and the manner in which the adolescent might dominate the household, the clinician can also inquire about the various responses and techniques parents have deployed in reaction to their child and the sequence of unfolding events during the course of development. Such information can provide the interviewer with a sense of the parents' personality and the manner in which they help to maintain the young person's problematic behaviors. In addition, rather than merely obtaining a listing of historically important events in the life of the child and the family, the clinician can try to explore the meaning of the events to the parent and the family "mythology" created about these events and milestones. This knowledge can help the clinician empathize with the adolescent's inner world and inform the clinician's understanding of the unfolding transference and countertransference.

# Peers

Knowledge of adolescents' friendship patterns, in individual and group settings, provides information about their capacity to sustain relationships and to experience intimacy and be empathic in such relationships; the kinds of roles they can take on in the group hierarchy; and the degree to which they can be mutually reliant and supportive rather than manipulative or exploitative with others. Do they have a best friend? Can they describe him or her with some nuance and in a manner that makes them seem real? Can they be dependent on the friend (e.g., ask for and take advice; give advice)? Are the activities they engage in real, and do these activities seem to generate real pleasure and move them toward maturity, or are they repetitive, with everyone "stuck" at the same developmental point? Do they have a range of friends that represent a split world (i.e., one with whom they feel close; a confidant or confidante who can listen to their woes but with whom they do not have a well-rounded relationship; and others, possibly the larger group, who they feel ridicule them or keep them at a distance)? Finally, inquiry into the nature of peer group activity is valuable for determining possible antisocial activity and alcohol or drug use. Some adolescents describe "hanging out" and "getting high" but are stumped if they are asked what they would do with friends if they did not "get high"; this response is indicative of the shallowness of these relationships and somewhat reminiscent of the parallel play of a very young child who has not yet moved on to establish reciprocal interactive patterns where each provides something toward a final, mutually constructed goal. The examples of different levels of BPO described earlier in this chapter illustrated how the severity of problems was manifested in friendships, especially how these problems distorted or prevented friendships, and indicate that the features that contribute to the adolescent's identity status are manifested in these relationships.

# Clinical Interviewing Process: The Structural Interview

Earlier in this chapter we described how procedures utilized in a general assessment of adolescents, such as behavioral rating scales and procedures and content gleaned from standardized semi-structured interviews, can contribute to the evaluation process. The procedures and the goals they permit the clinician to pursue are different from those that reflect the adolescent's identity status and the fundamental role this plays in understanding the personality organization and severity of the personality disorder. Here we will describe the joint use of the two procedures that are central to determining the adolescent's identity status and, hence, their level of BPO—the SI (Kernberg 1984; Yeomans et al. 2015) and the PAI (Selzer et al. 1987). The SI and PAI may be used to assess seven essential components of the adolescent's personality organization, several of which were described earlier (see Table 4–2): 1) cognitive features (ideas, memories, reality testing); 2) affects (e.g., impulses, desires); 3) self representation; 4) object representations (parents, close friends, therapists); 5) defenses; 6) empathic ability directed toward therapist; and 7) self-reflective functioning (capacity to observe the self). These procedures utilize the quality of the here-and-now interaction during the clinical interview, thus providing a suggestion of how the adolescent might react while engaging in TFP-A therapy itself.

The SI and PAI are quite different from typical structured and semi-structured interviews. The word *structure*, as used here, refers not to the characteristics of these measurement procedures but rather to the fact that the goal of the interviews is to assess the level and nature of the patient's internal psychological structure that is inferred from the degree of organization of their verbal responses. Therefore, the unfolding of the questioning is more open-ended than in a semi-structured interview and is guided in part by the adolescent's responses and the manner in the adolescent presents himself or herself. The SI format, in recognition of the fragmented and disorganized manner in which BPO individuals often construct their answers, does not expect the interview to proceed in a set pattern or direction. While the clinician has certain goals or endpoints in mind, how those are arrived at is open-ended and influenced by the quality and content of the adolescent's responses.

Things should make sense, so when responses are vague, when causal links are not clear or absent, or when there are gaps in the narrative, the clinician will utilize techniques such as clarification and confrontation, which are also deployed in the therapy process. Clarification is used to see whether the adolescent can understand why the other person might be confused by the adolescent's replies and whether a clearer, better organized response can be provided. Confrontation is utilized in the presence of contradictions, omissions, and inconsistencies in the adolescent's narrative. (see Chapter 6 for an expanded explanation of clarification and confrontation). It can then be observed whether the adolescent can reflect on the interviewer's comment, understand why his or her response seemed confusing, and reorganize his or her thoughts and present them in a coherent manner, rather than in the more chaotic manner that was first used; or whether, as is the case when there is identity diffusion, the adolescent becomes more anxious or defensive. However, despite the increase in anxiety, individuals with identity diffusion typically understand the basis of the interviewer's confusion and reorganize themselves and provide a clearer response. In contrast, in the presence of psychotic structure, they may not follow why the interviewer was confused and, more importantly, may become more disorganized in their thinking and talking as they try to respond further to the interviewer's inquiry.

The interviewer will often return to the adolescent's previous ideas and statements and ask questions that examine whether the adolescent can integrate and bring order to information that had originally been presented in a disjointed manner because of the impact of splitting-derived defenses. All the while the interviewer is attentive to the essential "channels of communication" (Caligor et al. 2018)—the young person's verbal and nonverbal behavior, manifestations of transference and countertransference—while also having in mind a representation of the range of normal adolescence so that these features can be viewed within a developmental context.

# Interview Procedures

The PAI focuses specifically on the moment-to-moment interaction between the clinician and the adolescent, while the SI offers a systematic method of inquiry that provides information about the seven components indicated at the opening of this section. The clinician may chose to smoothly integrate these two interviewing procedures to ask adolescents about their *problems* and thereby see whether they a) are able to demonstrate their awareness of what brought them to the clinician, b) show an ability to describe their problems in an organized way, and c) express their understanding of and feelings about their problems. These features of the SI and PAI expose the clinician to the adolescent's style of interacting with others. In so doing they get to observe adolescents' capacity to describe themselves and to see them reflect on self, others, and the responses they have made. Thus, the clinician becomes immersed in adolescents' display of their personality, is exposed to their defensive patterns, and experiences the presence of any pathological personality traits. These are features that contribute to evaluating level of identity formation and distinguishing between NPO and levels of BPO.

The PAI items might be used to open the interviewing process, and then its other elements can be interspersed as the interview proceeds. For example, at the outset the clinician can inquire about the adolescent's curiosity, awareness of his or her world, and anticipation of the treatment by asking, "What have you been told about this interview or meeting with me?" Then, the clinician can examine reflective functioning about an ongoing interpersonal interaction by asking at 10- to 15-minute intervals, "Now that we have been together for 15 minutes or so, how does what happened compare with your initial impressions, and what do you expect the rest of the meeting will be like?"; and, still later, "What have you learned about yourself, about me, and what do you imagine I have understood so far?" This can also set the stage for the feedback when the clinician will have the opportunity to present what he or she has learned and its implications. The PAI is well suited for adolescents because the clinician does not inquire about their private life, which may be examined in subsequent sessions. Furthermore, when the adolescent offers replies that are indicative of a preserved sense of self under these challenging interactions, it can help to differentiate between normal identity confusion and elements of identity diffusion. Finally, the PAI helps to assess the capacity of the adolescent to benefit from a psychotherapy, and especially TFP-A, because it taps such functions as attention, memory, reality testing, mentalization, and the capacity to sustain a working alliance under highly affective interactions. In particular, it very quickly gets to the adolescent's reflective ability, and by returning to this type of question several times, the clinician gets a sense of how the adolescent learns from and adapts to this very novel situation that requires talking to an adult in what must be a very unfamiliar way.

The SI quickly draws attention to the adolescents' awareness of their symptoms and their understanding of their problems by asking an essential question such as "What brings you to this meeting" or "What is your understanding of why we are meeting?" Subsequent questions might include "Are you consenting to be here?" "What would you say are the nature of your difficulties?" "What would you say are your parents' perceptions of your difficulties?" and "What is your idea about therapy, and what are you expecting from it?" Thus, the interview progresses toward the exploration of adolescents' awareness and understanding of their problems—do they wish for help with how they feel and act and wish things were different in their life? (That is, do they express a wish for treatment, and are they motivated for change?) Effective TFP-A with young people is greatly enhanced if they can be helped to identify something that they hope to get out of their treatment.

The next essential question, "Tell me about yourself," provides insight into the young person's identity status. While the previous question(s) that asked for a description of the problem may be difficult for some and elicit somewhat disjointed answers depending on BPO level, many still find it easier to describe their problem than to describe themselves or others. The former typically refers to overt behaviors that involve direct interactions with their world and about which they are receiving feedback, often negative. Sometimes a difference in the response to each of these questions can be quite informative. Their responses also inform about their reality testing—that is, are their internal representations producing distorted perceptions of self or others, or interactions? This path of inquiry can be expanded by asking adolescents to describe, for example, their parents and best friends, as well as their religion and ethnic background; how they see themselves physically; and how they deal with changing events (Kernberg et al. 2000).

In addition to providing information about personality structure, including defenses and coping style, quality of self and other representations, and identity confusion/diffusion, this interview procedure provides information about the adolescent's mastery of important developmental tasks that have prognostic significance. The interview also provides information about their approach to (or avoidance) of school/work, peers, sexuality/intimacy, morality, separation, and their ability to develop and start to carry out future plans. In addition, it allows for the pursuit of the individualization of treatment goals (discussed below) as an attempt is made, together with the adolescent, to identify his or her personal goals, as distinct from the parents', that will serve as a motivation to pursue treatment.

Finally, the clinician asks the adolescent if there was anything left out of the interview—anything the adolescent thought the clinician should know about or anything the adolescent wanted to ask the clinician. This type of question may have different meaning depending on level of pathology. That is, an NPO youngster is more likely to view the clinician as potentially helpful and might be more inclined to add to the interview with his or her own questions; a low-BPO adolescent may be more likely to view the clinician as potentially malevolent and so would seek to avoid further engagement.

## Goals

The types of goals that adolescents express can be quite variable and may reflect very different elements in the developmental process depending on the age of the adolescent, but they are typically quite meaningful and informative. For example, Anna, the 19-year-old whose case was discussed earlier, in response to a question about what she hoped to get from the consultation and from her therapy, offered as her goal the opportunity to be able to live with her parents who want to "kick me out." It would appear incongruous that this was the goal of an adolescent who described and displayed (in individual and joint meetings) animosity toward her mother despite their expressions of synchronous smiling and laughing. While this may have been her goal, a goal of the assessment was to move from a behavioral attainment (i.e., living under the same roof with her mother) to a clarification and understanding of underlying nonconscious factors that are related to the goal. For example, after Anna spoke a bit about her mother and their relationship, she spontaneously described her unfaithfulness to her boyfriend but stated it was unrelated to her relationship with her mother. The clinician was very *active* (i.e., did not remain silent or let Anna's dismissal of her association remain unnoticed), confronting her minimization of this association, and suggested that Anna may have been describing a conflict with sustaining intimacy, with both mother and boyfriend. She looked wide-eyed at the clinician and agreed while expressing amazement. In effect, the clarified and transformed goal was to understand Anna's difficulty with intimacy, which was interfering with her maintaining stability and closeness with people she cared about; this could eventually allow for an exploration of her attachment patterns and the defensive operations associated with them. Of course, this approach could be one contributor toward her goal of being able to eventually live with her parents, but it would also have a much broader significance. Similarly, for a younger adolescent who expressed the goal of wanting to have more friends, the more profound goal became recognizing, understanding, and doing something about his frequent lying, which was interfering with his ability to maintain friendships.

# Clinical Illustrations of Structural Interviewing

The examples of NPO and levels of BPO provided earlier in this chapter were based on evidence provided by the use of SI and the other TFP-A techniques described in this manual. Here we present two brief vignettes that give more of a sense of the adolescent's direct replies to the SI and PAI inquiries and provide a flavor of the individual's internal structure.

The first interview provides a sense of how the SI can offer a window into what is meant by underlying structure. For this 16-year-old girl, the nonspecific nature of the SI questioning exposed her poorly developed internal structure. Her begging for questions is an indication of how, for her, a structured interview would have been a very different experience and therefore indicates the value of the SI format for examining internal structure and assessing personality organization.

## Case 2: Amy

Amy, a 16-year-old, was interviewed during her third psychiatric hospitalization. She made a dramatic entrance to the conference room. She had dyed hair, wore dark lipstick, and was smiling and laughing as she said hello to those whom she already knew who were attending the case conference and seemed happy to greet those whom she did not know. She easily transitioned to explaining her understanding of the case conference and then described why she thought she was in the hospital (i.e., cutting, suicidal intention) and quickly began to talk about her mother, although she was not asked to do so. However, when the interviewer asked her, "Tell me about yourself," she reacted with panic, had difficulty remaining in her seat, did not look at or address the interviewer, and pleaded loudly toward the other conference attendees that they should ask her questions. She said she was used to questions, and could respond to those, but could not just talk about herself. In effect, she was not able to organize her own thoughts and construct a response that reflected how she saw herself; she instead required others to provide a structure for her by asking questions.

The next vignette describes a young adolescent boy with a low BPO that is reflected in his fear of annihilation. The SI and the use of clarification and confrontation provided an understanding of how his aggression was a defense against this fear and the manner in which his paranoid style was active at such moments. In addition, he showed different response patterns to requests to describe his problem and to describe himself. His response to the interviewer's interventions suggested he had some potential to work toward understanding and integrating the roles of victim and victimizer and his use of projection. It is important to be able to recognize an adolescent's strengths as well as his or her compromised functioning.

## Case 3: Harry

Harry, a very intelligent 13-year-old, was interviewed at a case conference during his fifth hospitalization, all of which had taken place in the last 18 months. The reasons for each hospitalization typically stemmed from his verbally threatening and physically assaultive behaviors. These ranged from comments about wanting to kill someone to actually stabbing a teacher with a pencil. His aggressive behavior first occurred at 18 months of age, directed at a younger sibling. Currently, the people in his life are frightened of any threats he makes, and his parents' behavior has ranged from avoidance to long-standing expressions of wanting "to be rid of him." He had been participating in once-weekly individual psychotherapy for about 18 months with his current therapist, who likes him. Some of the hospital staff who had contact with him across several of the hospitalizations also reported experiencing positive feelings toward him, including sympathy, apparently derived from negative countertransferential feelings toward his parents. After he was introduced to the observers at the conference, he replied softly, in the affirmative, when he was asked whether he wanted to know who the other attendees were. So, at this point, what was known is that this is a youngster with a long history of aggressive, assaultive behavior that seemed to be increasing in lethality and that he could not control, and that was not being controlled by a variety of interventions, including psychotropic medication; parental relationships that indicated significant problems with the attachment process; some potential wish for interpersonal connections; and a capacity to be liked by some. The system also suggested the possibility of splitting, between parents and various therapists.

Harry was asked to express his understanding of why he was in the hospital. He vaguely described some of his aggressive behavior, that he was doing "rude" things. Harry then went on to describe being attacked several times by another youngster at a day-treatment facility that he had been attending. The description of his behavior was vague and superficial with a rapid externalization and projection of blame onto other children, suggesting a dyad with a division between a victimized self and a bad, hostile, destructive other, in which the former was perceived as good within the context of an angry, aggressive relation with the latter. As he got deeper into this explanation, he seemed to the interviewer to be presenting an automatized description of his behavior and his plight, as if he were offering a repetitive script that incorporated what he had heard others say about him or to him regarding what he must do to improve. In effect, his description of his problem was boring and seemed rehearsed and superficial. He made little eye contact, which he acknowledged later in the interview. Thus, he was able to offer some commentary on the overt behavior that had led to his hospitalization, but to this point he appeared somewhat detached from his narrative and showed little insight about why he acted as he did.

When Harry was then asked, "Tell me about yourself," he slumped in his chair, his gaze avoidance increased, he said very little, and, even more informatively, his attempt to express something was very incomplete and disorganized. He did not present anything that provided any information about him, how he saw himself, or how he thought others saw him. These features of his self-description, as well as its contrast to his description of his problems, despite those deficiencies, raised the question of identity diffusion. He then reorganized himself a bit by utilizing projection, resuming his complaints about the boy who had been attacking him. He said the boy was "delusional" and went on to describe the boy's unjustified fantasy that had led him to attack Harry. Because of his introduction of this term, Harry was then asked if we could return to talking about him, and he was asked whether he had any "delusions" and, if so, to describe them. He quickly spoke about his belief that others would attack him. The interviewer commented that he sounded as if he were often fearful. Harry agreed and spoke further about his fear and his aggression. The interviewer then said to Harry, "Tell me if I followed you correctly—you thought the other boy believed you were a threat to him and so he attacked you, and you often believe people want to harm you and so you attack them." He said that was accurate, paused, and then began to make eye contact with the interviewer, who said, "So, is it possible that you attack people because you believe they want to destroy you and it makes you feel safe if you destroy them first?" He sighed and said, "Finally, someone understands." This sequence illustrates Harry's paranoid orientation and associated defensive structure that supports his aggression. Also, his response to the intervention suggests he has some potential to work toward understanding and integrating the roles of victim and victimizer and his use of projection as a way of dealing with his fear of annihilation.

The appendix to this chapter presents segments of a more extended interview that illustrates many of the SI, PAI and TFP-A techniques with a hospitalized 16-year-old boy who showed significant narcissistic pathology.

# Feedback

As with any feedback after an evaluation, parents will expect to be told what is wrong (i.e., what is causing their child's problems for which they initiated this evaluation and they can do). The adolescent who is being evaluated may have similar questions but may dread or not seek an answer. These expectations exist even when the evaluation was initiated by someone other than the parents, such as the school or legal authorities. As indicated at various points in this manual, the feedback can lead to a sequential approach to understanding the adolescent and treatment recommendations. That is, when there is a severe co-occurring problem such as drug/alcohol use disorder, eating disorder, or OCD, an initial intervention may be recommended to reduce the potential interfering impact of these disorders on the TFP-A treatment of the PD. Also, when there is severe underachievement reflected in a refusal to do schoolwork, which typically has a constant impact on the life of the family and the adolescent, a preliminary plan may be worked out among school, parent, and adolescent in an attempt to stabilize school functioning. Otherwise, school issues and demands of school and parents may constantly intrude into the psychotherapy. This is not to say that the therapy will ignore the adolescent's struggle with meeting this important demand of his or her life, but, as discussed in Chapter 5, it is best for the treatment if a frame is established that attempts to address and contain known, historically disruptive features in the adolescent's life.

If the assessment indicates the presence of a PD, and if there is also a comorbid disorder, as is often the case when a PD is present, it will be incumbent on the clinician to discuss the Axis I disorder(s) and the PD. The comorbid disorder will typically include features that have been apparent to the parents and to the adolescent and that most likely prompted the evaluation. For the parents and the adolescents to have a full and meaningful understanding of the assessment findings, it is necessary for the explanation of the diagnosis to show an understanding of these presenting problems—how they are accounted for—and why they are manifested as they have been—their type of presentation in different settings (e.g., at school, with peers, at home).

Parents' expectations and wishes from the feedback may vary widely. Some have the attitude that they will just have their child appear for treatment and some solution will magically occur. Others will attentively take in the feedback as they would with an evaluation from any doctor, and their compliance will be determined by their needs and personality type. Still others may have clear beliefs about what is going on with their child and may have an investment in maintaining that belief—whether it is to see it as more benign or to attribute it to a cause that leaves them feeling vindicated or blameless. Regardless of the situation, when a PD is part of the diagnosis, it is essential that the clinician explain the nature of PD to the parents and, in particular, clarify how this diagnosis helps clinician and parents understand their child's problems and informs the choice of treatment approach. For example, many adolescents will display anxiety, but it will range in severity and be manifested in different ways. When a PD is implicated, the explanation broadens to go beyond general anxiety disorder, phobia, or even panic, forms that many families have some familiarity with, to illustrate how such a conceptualization helps in understanding and treating the problem.

With Harry, this understanding moved from a long-standing concentration on his aggression and assaultiveness to a depiction of his extreme fearfulness (paranoid defenses and projection), his worry about being attacked and destroyed (fear of annihilation), and his counter-phobic behavioral style of attacking first. With Anna, a first step involved identifying the role anxiety was playing in her life and in her family's. This had received minor attention in her previous hospitalizations and treatment because, understandably, attention was drawn to her aggressive, defiant, and often dangerous behaviors. These behaviors still needed to be kept in sight and incorporated into contract planning. However, a significant dimension was added to everyone's understanding by explaining how her particular personality problem, derived from basic issues of insecure attachment, led to difficulty maintaining closeness and intimacy (which part of her wanted) while also supporting her fear of rejection and abandonment. It could then be understood that her panic about closeness and fear of abandonment were intertwined, promoted her erratic behavior and extreme inconsistency in her relationships, and her difficulty in being dependent and fully accepting help in previous therapies. It then followed that the treatment ultimately should be focused not solely on her oppositional and antisocial behaviors, or even her anxiety, but on how her sense of self that emanated from her disordered attachment representations drove her actions. This type of focus promotes an integrative understanding of the adolescent's symptomatology into a framework that offers meaning to a heretofore disparate and confusing picture. When this occurs, a recommendation of TFP-A as a treatment choice to the adolescent and parents can make sense, especially for youngsters who have experienced previously unsuccessful treatments that tended to focus on ameliorating the overt behavioral features associated with the BPO structure, such as anxiety or acting-out behaviors.

It may also be necessary to revisit with some parents their understanding of their child's disorder. Because a PD is an inherently inferential diagnosis, it can be difficult for some parents, even those who are very intelligent, successful, and well read, to grasp. For example, the low-BPO adolescent described earlier in this chapter presented a complicated picture. He seemed depressed, at times had suicidal ideation, and behaved in a manner that fit descriptions of oppositional defiant behavior, and some knowledgable friends even suggested to the parents that perhaps he was "on the spectrum." Psychiatric consultation led to trials of antidepressants, medication that focused on ADHD, and a low dose of atypical antipsychotic medication because of the paranoid, possibly psychotic quality to his thinking during moments of rage. None of these were effective, but they were important attempts to help with his behavioral disruption. The explanation to him and his parents (given at separate times and repeated when necessary) sought in everyday language to provide an understanding of his narcissism organized at a low-BPO level—that is, the rage associated with the narcissism; his poor self-image that made him sensitive to any anticipated negative comments, leading to avoidance of schoolwork; his compensatory grandiosity that made him disparage everyone else (including his therapist) and maintain a demand of greatness of himself that could not be achieved and affected his ability sustain his effort; his paranoid fear of others promoting his isolation from friends and family; a deeper neediness that prevented him from giving and taking from parents because of a fear of dependency; and his need for omnipotent control to maintain a fragile coping style. Even more concretely, it is not that all parties are simply told that the adolescent is paranoid; rather, it is noted that in his descriptions he typically presents himself as a victim and that he avoids others whom he sees as against him. This is a perspective that offers understanding to his behavior with family, peers, and teachers. Therefore, a goal might be to examine his conception of others more closely because it would serve his goal of wanting to be happier. With schoolwork, the issue was not that he lacked the intelligence to succeed, but rather that his excellent ability was not allowed to be displayed because his current goal that he must be better than everyone led him to withdraw from the contest. A treatment goal might be to arrive at a new basis for self-evaluation, one that was neither overinflated nor diminished. The attempt is to arrive at realistic goals. These explanations of course would not make his refusal to do schoolwork or his anger and oppositional behavior any more acceptable, but they would provide an integrative understanding that would make sense to everyone and that supported the framework of TFP-A as a treatment approach.

# Conclusion

The determination of the presence of PDs in adolescents should occur in the context of a comprehensive evaluation that assesses comorbid psychiatric disorders such as mood, anxiety, and conduct disorders, as well as academic and cognitive functioning. Developmental history, family functioning, and peer relations should also be examined.

Pharmacological intervention for any mood, anxiety, or behavioral problems should be considered.

Structural interviewing contributes to the identification of identity status and distinguishing between identity crisis and identity diffusion. Diagnosing identity status is essential for determining the presence of a PD.

Identifying severity of PD, defined as level of BPO, is an important goal of the assessment procedure. Distinguishing among NPO and high, mid-, or low BPO informs both diagnosis and treatment planning and expectations. These distinctions among NPO and the different levels of BPO are based on the adolescent's organization of self and other representations; defenses; aggression; and moral functioning. Reality testing is also assessed.

Feedback to the adolescent and parents attempts to offer an explanation that provides an understanding of how the behaviors that were of concern and that prompted the evaluation, and that might seem quite disparate, are viewed in an integrated manner best explained by a diagnosis of PD. The treatment recommended can then be seen as following from this diagnostic conclusion.

# Appendix: Extended Interview With Richard, a 16-Year-Old With Narcissistic Features

The interview took place in an inpatient hospital, where Richard (fictional name) had recently been admitted for depression.

## Excerpt 1

The therapist opens the interview by asking Richard what he knew and expected about their meeting and then goes on to ask him to tell about himself. Richard attempts to avoid answering and seeks to seize control of the direction of the discussion. The therapist's comments illustrate how this interview format focuses on the "here and now" and emphasizes the point by saying, *"We are going to talk about what is going on right now in this interaction."*

The therapist initially asks Richard what he knows about her and this meeting. He comments that he was told that the therapist is a "senior executive." She asks Richard what he makes of this. He replies: *"It shows that obviously my case is of some importance for the team....And that maybe there's something about me you want to hear and maybe that you've had dealings with people like me before, well, I hope...is this true?"* Thus, Richard quickly displays the haughty, sometimes arrogant quality that is evident throughout the interview and striking in the video. Yet, he ends his comment with a note of uncertainty. The therapist asks about the uncertainty reflected in Richard's comments: *"So, you have doubts about your reflections, if your reflections are right or wrong. Do you think you're right?"* Richard says: *"Oh, I think I'm right...Yes."* Then the therapist confronts him about this contradiction: *"Yes, so why were you asking me if this is right?"*

Shortly after this exchange, the therapist says: *"I was interested in who you are, and...so I wanted to hear about how you feel about coming and interviewing... it's not a regular meeting...Saturday morning."* Rather than replying directly to the therapist's question, Richard responds with a question:

RICHARD: First, well, let me ask you a question. What have you heard about me? Obviously you heard something because you're coming here and you're talking to me and making a special effort.
THERAPIST: The therapy team wanted to hear some of my impressions, and I will be giving feedback to you too later in the interview.
RICHARD: Well, I'd like some...not feedback of what I am saying right now, but feedback of what you've heard from the team already.
THERAPIST: Oh, you know, in that respect, what we are going to talk about is what is going right now in this interaction."

# Excerpt 2

The therapist is cognizant of what Richard is saying as well as alert to his behavior and other expressions of emotions (e.g., smile, cough, somatization) throughout the interview, which are inquired about. In addition, although detours occur, the therapist does not lose sight of the goal of the interview component, which is to allow Richard to describe himself.

The discussion in the first excerpt continues for a while, so Richard comments: *"So you are not allowed to tell me?"* The therapist points out that there was a contradiction in Richard's comments: if he thought she was a "senior executive," who would be giving her orders? The therapist, picking up on Richard's comment and wording, follows this thread:

THERAPIST: I have to follow protocols and not make up rules? What is interesting is that I was going to tell you how we were going to proceed today, but you are telling me that I'm not allowed to, right?
RICHARD: No, I'm saying that...
THERAPIST: You're smiling, what is it that makes you smile?
RICHARD: What makes me smile?

Richard goes on to review by repeating his request and notes that the therapist said they would be talking about what was occurring in their meeting, not what the team might have said about him. The therapist concurs that he understood her correctly, and Richard notes that it would make him comfortable if he knew what came before, reflecting a paranoid component.

RICHARD: I wanna hear what happened prior to this meeting right now so I know where you're coming from.

THERAPIST: I think we have a disagreement in perspective...you want to talk about what I knew about you before I got here from what I discussed with the team. You are interested in that, and what I am saying is I'm not doing that because I am going to focus my interview with you on you and what we are discussing right now. So...I wanted to hear about how you see yourself, how you describe yourself, and we can begin with that. So suppose you have to introduce yourself to me. I have to say that I really don't know you except that you are here, but I'm not sure why you are here, at this moment, I want to see who you are. I want you to introduce yourself, and we'll see who you are. Agree?

RICHARD: Yes.

THERAPIST: So now we have agreement. [Later she asks Richard to describe friends and parents.]

# Excerpt 3

Thus, the therapist maintains the structure of the interview; is alert to Richard's defensive maneuvers, conscious and unconscious, and comments on them so that the purpose of the interview is not lost; and has brought Richard back to that point and will continue to do so when necessary. The value of the SI and PAI is illustrated in this excerpt because the patient ultimately provides a very valuable description of self that captures an important essence of his PD.

RICHARD: So I will introduce myself as...I will describe myself as a person who is intelligent...who can understand people very well, and who generally can see through the images that people try to convey, and I would say that overall, I am very different than other people, I believe.

Richard is distracted by another child's voice, and Richard and the therapist briefly talk about his hospitalization experience and the fact that he has been there for 4 days.

RICHARD: Hmm...It's very humiliating. I know it's hospitalization. I know that it's designed for treatment, but I also know that I, I believe that there should be two adolescent units, one for high-functioning people and one for low functioning.

THERAPIST: I think we got a little side tracked?

RICHARD: Yes, but that's just my take on the situation.

THERAPIST: Yeah, so you were describing—introducing yourself—to me, and you got distracted and stopped this.

RICHARD: So, hmm…I would say that my personality allows me to . . . understand people in a way that nobody else can…and that allows me to do certain things.

THERAPIST: Can you give me some examples of that?

At various times the therapist asks Richard for concrete examples, which is indicative of the fact that many of his answers that might ordinarily seem informative are not. In addition, the therapist offers an interpretation of Richard's tendency to talk in "generalities," that his earlier comments indicate that he is "somebody who is very interested in power," and that he may be trying to exert power in this interview.

RICHARD: I mean in a short period of time and with a little bit more bonding, I can create connections with people that no one else can in such a rapid time and with such a strong connection.

THERAPIST: How would you describe that? What is it that you have that makes people feel attracted, interested, or drawn to you?

RICHARD: Well, I'm saying that on the outside, I'm very personable and very…talkative …but on the inside…everything I say has a meaning and purpose…everything I say is used to achieve a certain goal.

THERAPIST: Would you say that you're achieving the goal right now, of describing yourself? Because that was the purpose of our talk. I asked that you introduce yourself to me right now. Well, does that mean that you are achieving a goal right now?

RICHARD: Oh well, I am a very difficult person to describe…maybe yes, maybe I would say that I have achieved my goal. That's a very interesting question that you posed. Would you say that I achieved my goal?

THERAPIST: You seem to be in the process of it…I have to say that you communicate straightforwardly, that everything you say is meaningful, that you describe yourself that way on the outside, but on the inside, which is here, does it apply?

RICHARD: I would say that on the inside, it doesn't apply.

Richard goes on to say that inside the hospital he feels like "I'm being arrested from myself" and that he feels distant from the person he is on the outside, like a "dethroned king." In response to the interviewer, he indicates that he "controls the atmosphere" around him and can "just tell" that he has this effect. The therapist confronts this construct and eventually his lying, by clearly indicating when she does not believe him.

THERAPIST: You know that here you are talking in generalities?

RICHARD: You want specifics?

THERAPIST: Yeah, something specific…Would that be possible? Because here you are saying that you are somebody who is very interested in power…and here you may also be making attempts with me to be like the throned king. So do you think I could have doubts about your power if I told you that it's not possible?…Do you understand that I could think that?

(*Richard coughs.*)

THERAPIST: I made you cough?

RICHARD: I laughed…

THERAPIST: A laugh? I know that it's not….I don't sense that I…I don't get it.

RICHARD: I found it amusing.

THERAPIST: Amusing, eh. Do you have the feeling that I am laughing at you?

RICHARD: No.

They go on to talk about lies he has acknowledged he has told others, including peers and hospital staff. He expresses the idea that he could feel guilty about that. The therapist demonstrates the importance of openly confronting the antisocial element she detects in this narcissistic young person.

RICHARD: But they are still lies, aren't they? Despite how I feel.

THERAPIST: Did they catch you?

RICHARD: Yes. Despite…

THERAPIST: If they didn't catch you, you would still feel bad?

RICHARD: Yes. Despite how I feel.

THERAPIST: Yes or no?

RICHARD: Yes, I said yes.

THERAPIST: See, in this I don't believe you so much. This time I don't believe you because I look at your face and you look triumphant about not being caught. You are smart enough to get it done, no?

RICHARD: I'd still have to live with the guilt.

THERAPIST: Guilt, what guilt?

RICHARD: Guilt! That I broke the rules and now I have to live with that.

THERAPIST: How do you recognize that emotion in you?

RICHARD: Guilt usually builds up in me in the form of anxiety.

THERAPIST: Anxiety. Can you tell me what your experience is?

RICHARD: Stomach pain.

THERAPIST: And does it hurt?

RICHARD: It hurts very much, but I still feel a sensation in my head and in my stomach and I get tired. That's why I have to be very careful about the mistakes that I make. I have to make sure that I don't do anything that will have detrimental effects to my mental and physical health.

THERAPIST: Given the fact that you were smiling at me, it gives me the sense like you are saying you have gotten away with murder, and it gives the sense of triumph, especially since you think of yourself as a king.

Richard is asked to describe friends and parents. The therapist then asks Richard to offer his reflections on their meeting.

> THERAPIST: We have spent almost 40 minutes now. Have you learned any-
> thing about me, since you said at the beginning that you had almost
> like antennae. How would you describe talking with me?
> RICHARD: Well then again, you didn't do much talking did you? I was the
> one who did most of the talking and you did the listening.

The therapist then provides feedback to Richard, offering her impressions in a systematic, concrete manner that Richard understands. They then talk about what he has gotten from the interview.

> THERAPIST: Ok, we have to stop unfortunately…and thank you.
> RICHARD: Yes, it was very pleasant. Did you get anything out of this?
> THERAPIST: I think I got to know you, and I gave you my feedback. What
> about you, what do you think?
> RICHARD: I think that from your position, yes, a lot did happen here. You
> were able to extract a lot of information out of me, maybe not from
> what I've said, but maybe from my tone or little sentences or phrases
> that came out of me, that maybe I didn't want to say or that…despite
> whether I wanted to say it or not, it still says a lot about me, just from
> normal interactions. Yes, I think you did get a lot from me, you did
> get a lot.
> THERAPIST: And what about you?
> RICHARD: What about me?
> THERAPIST: Hmm…Would you say that you learned something about your-
> self?
> RICHARD: I don't know, I don't know if there's anything about me that I don't
> already know.

# Observations on Interview

The interviewer demonstrated the use of several TFP-A techniques, including clarification, confrontation, and interpretation. Limit setting was used frequently so as not to lose control of the direction of the interview while pursuing the attempt to have the patient describe himself. The therapist was also alert to nonverbal expressions by the patient and integrated the information derived from them into the discussion.

Regarding diagnosis, this interview demonstrated that someone as young as 16 years could be characterized by clear narcissistic PD with antisocial features organized at a borderline level. He displayed his underlying vulnerability, expressed at one moment somewhat despairingly as the dethroned king. There was also the humiliation of being in the hospital that he attempted to defend against by trying to take control of the interview and suggesting that the patients should be split and that he would belong in the superior unit. His attempt to compensate by being the powerful one in charge of the interview was identified and labeled by the interviewer and coupled with limit setting.

The patient expressed features of a pathological grandiose self constructed to protect against this vulnerable self. He described himself as intelligent and able to skillfully read others. This empathic ability, which is basic to moral functioning, was not used to that end or in a compassionate way, but was enlisted to manipulate, control, and exploit others. Thus, his mentalization was compromised by the projection of the devalued self. His antisocial picture was completed by his lying.

Finally, despite several attempts by the interviewer, he did not really offer a complex, integrated picture of himself or peers.

He wanted reassurance and comfort but did not allow himself to truly take a dependent position and show his need for support. Not shown in these excerpts was his description of asking his mother for support, but by manipulating her to lie and cheat on his behalf.

# CHAPTER 5

# Establishing the Treatment Frame and Parent Collaboration

**THE CONTRACTING PHASE** is considered the first tactic in Transference-Focused Psychotherapy for Adolescents (TFP-A), and treatment tactics are the tasks the therapist must attend to before beginning the treatment. The goal is to create a frame that will allow opportunities for adolescents to engage themselves in their responsibilities, appropriate developmental tasks, and adaptive behaviors while experiencing a sense of decision making and liberty, and to obtain the parents' collaboration.

## Establishing the Contract

There are eight aspects in establishing a contract that must be considered: 1) agreeing on a common understanding of the adolescent's problems in terms of personality disorders and "identity diffusion"; 2) educating the adolescent about TFP-A and his or her role; 3) encouraging the active participation of the adolescent in the contract setting; 4) establishing a "safe" frame for the treatment; 5) anticipating and preventing forms of resistance that could threaten continuation of the treatment; 6) beginning to rework maladaptive functioning through behavioral activation; 7) agreeing to engage with developmental tasks; and 8) establishing the basis of collaboration with parents.

# Agreeing on a Common Understanding of the Adolescent's Problems

The feedback to the parent and the adolescent will partly depend on the age of the adolescent. With all ages we suggest a joint feedback so that adolescent and parent know that they are receiving the same information. Older adolescents may also have separate feedback to approach any questions they or the therapist believe require confidentiality immediately into the process, and such a meeting quickly begins transitioning the process to individual psychotherapy.

Findings from the assessment should be integrated with the presenting problems so that parents and adolescent recognize that the therapist has not lost sight of what brought them for treatment and that their initial concerns are being addressed. This could include comments about mood, anxiety, behavioral problems, and recommendations for additional testing (e.g., assessments for learning disability, and attention-deficit disorder; medical evaluations) or pharmacology evaluations.

It is necessary to communicate our understanding of the adolescent's problems and recommendation of treatment to both the adolescent and his or her parents. The therapist has to attempt to enhance the parents' understanding of the adolescent, the nature and seriousness of their child's difficulties, why TFP-A therapy is being recommended, and how it will approach the problem. We encourage parents to look for examples to understand how the personality pathology of the adolescent is the main cause of their discomfort and the difficulties they observe. In effect, the object relations model is explained in a concrete manner. For example, the anger parents describe and the adolescent acknowledges can be explained in terms of how the adolescent sees himself or herself or others at a certain moment; that the situation may be inducing extreme, uncomfortable and unmanageable affect; and that what is occurring is an ineffective way to manage the understandable discomfort. The TFP-A therapy tries to offer another way of handling these internal events (feelings, thoughts) so that both behaviors and feelings may change.

It is also explained that TFP-A is not a treatment that offers direct advice; the therapist will not generally tell the adolescent what to do (although more specific, concrete interventions will be offered in moments of danger, crisis, and significantly poor judgment). The therapist may comment, "Together, we will try to help you learn about yourself," and discuss why it is thought that would be helpful for the particular problem. A comment such as this also provides a message about process and expectations to those parents whose message to the therapist is, "Just fix it." In addition to talking about pathology, we help them understand and think about the consequences and likely evolution of the difficulties if there is no intervention and the adolescent does not receive help.

# Educating the Adolescent About TFP-A and His or Her Role

The discussion about the contract lays out the roles and responsibilities of the therapist, the adolescent, and the parents. Adolescents will differ greatly, as a function of age, sophistication, experience, and personality organization, in their ability to imagine how therapy works and envision how they are to play their role. Therefore, they will need to be educated about the therapy process, to move beyond the frame. This is not a single "lecture" but an ongoing process as the therapy unfolds and specific roadblocks are encountered.

For example, the importance of regular attendance is not merely couched as another rule they, as the child, must obey. Instead, it can be explained that they, like others their age and older, have an inner world; their thoughts and feelings have an impact on how they go about their life— school, friends, alone time, family.

> The kind of therapy I am suggesting for us to do believes that one important way to help you achieve your goals that brought you here is to explore that inner world so you can understand why you feel a certain way, how those feelings affect why you do or don't do something. So, if you didn't feel like coming to therapy one day, that would be something we could talk about. Some young people might feel that they shouldn't tell me; that I'll think they're bad and not like them; or that I'll tell their parents. Rather, that feeling of not wanting to come and talk has important meaning about what you might be feeling, about something that is bothering you, including something that is happening in our meetings, and if we could talk about that maybe you would understand yourself better. It's like a heavy burden—if you share the load it's easier to carry. You may have others kinds of thoughts that you believe, if expressed, would be embarrassing and make you feel foolish, and while I understand how unpleasant a feeling that can be, I would encourage you to share those kinds of thoughts as well.

In effect, the therapist is offering a "pre-interpretation interpretation" to explain the process and prepare for later interpretation proper about content, defense, transference, and so forth. It is done initially in a somewhat concrete way that utilizes imagery (sharing the load) and normalizes the process by making some issues universal, covering many ages and not just adolescence in particular, in an empathic context that shows awareness and appreciation for the adolescent's discomfort and anguish.

Procedures such as these, if not understood or utilized by the adolescent, may indicate that he or she is not a good candidate for TFP-A. The therapist can then work with the adolescent and parents toward finding a therapy that might be more amenable to their needs and abilities.

# Encouraging the Active Participation of the Adolescent

Adolescents with personality disorders find coping with the developmental challenges of adolescence difficult and consequently struggle to function effectively at home, at school, and with their peer group. Their experiences in childhood have failed to prepare them for the challenges of adolescence, and neurobiological changes have overstrained the capacity for organizing or strengthening their defensive or adaptive system. These youth face particular challenges, because the developmental task for adolescent and young people is to separate and individuate from parents and to develop a degree of autonomy. Adolescents with borderline personality disorder often attempt to become autonomous in the absence of key capacities to exercise autonomy safely, which increases anxiety in parents and professionals alike.

Encouraging active participation of the adolescent in the contract setting stage presents challenges but is highly valuable. Promoting active engagement in decision making can be done by outlining treatment options with the adolescent, highlighting the consequences of certain behaviors or choices and evaluating the benefits and disadvantages of behavior change.

## Case 1: Jacob

Jacob, a 13-year-old, is brought to the clinic by his parents after his school threatened to expel him because he physically and seriously assaulted another student. In spite of above-average intellectual ability, he is failing at school and has a long history of oppositional behavior at school and at home. At home, his parents are at a loss as to how to deal with his swings from being oppositional, provocative, and argumentative to being stubbornly silent and passive-aggressive, or, at other times, overly dependent, infantile, and submissive. They are also concerned about the extent to which he is bullying his younger brother. In addition, he is eating uncontrollably and never seems satisfied, and as a result he is becoming increasingly overweight. In terms of his early history, his mother describes him as having been a demanding and hypersensitive baby. Her first impression of him at birth was that there was something in the way that he looked at her that evoked a fear in her that he would suck her dry.

The first meeting with Jacob takes place in the presence of the parents. Both of them are angry at Jacob's oppositional attitude and lack of concern about them and his brother, and his tendency to exaggerate minor faults or reveal potentially shameful things that his brother does, like "stealing cookies and eating them at night." Their despair reached the level of sharing in front of Jacob their wish to get rid of him as soon as he turns 18. They are coming to treatment because they do not want to feel that they are "bad parents." They are hoping, with not much conviction, that therapy can reroute an already dysfunctional path.

Alone with Jacob, the therapist listens to Jacob relate his own perception of the problem, which is highly infiltrated with projection and denial of his responsibilities. After taking notice of his predictable refusal to come to therapy, the therapist engages Jacob in an open discussion on how to solve the problem of being compelled to come to therapy because of his parents' decision and authority over him, and his desire to stay mute and sabotage the treatment.

THERAPIST: I understand that as long as you do not see any advantage to coming here, there is no way either your parents or me will succeed in making you benefit from the treatment.

JACOB: I will come, otherwise they will continue to treat me like "garbage," but no one will force me to talk.

THERAPIST: I am glad that we are on the same wavelength; that is exactly what I am saying, what I meant by saying no one will succeed in making you benefit from treatment. But on the other hand, the two of us are stuck. You do not want to be forced to do things that you do not choose to do, and I understand that well. But from my side, I can't accept to offer a "dummy" treatment in the sense that the two of us know that it will not work.

JACOB: Yes, you can! Or you can tell my parents that it will not work.

THERAPIST: Yes, this is a possibility, but it will only solve my problem, not yours. You will still have to face your problem that you can't tolerate to be forced to do things that you do not want to and therefore have to rely on a "childish" method like not talking, though powerful I admit, because I gather that you have pride in yourself and would, in other circumstances, choose another means to express your strength, but you can't. When it happens, it is too strong.

JACOB: Hmm…hmm.

THERAPIST: Would you say that we have discovered something important here…that you have been experiencing that problem over and over, with your parents, at school, with friends? You can't tolerate to be forced to do things [here the therapist did not want to engage into a confrontation about the origin of this perception], and it puts you into a delicate situation to get into an argument either with adults, who will impose their authority, or with friends, who also want to have their chance to impose their choice, so they may let you down

> more often than not, or may make you lose pride in yourself because
> you can't argue, can't negotiate, can't compromise.
> JACOB: Hmm…hmm.
> THERAPIST: Would you say that if you had to decide yourself to come to therapy
> it would be an important issue to discuss, to look at, to be helped with.
> JACOB: Yes.
> THERAPIST: So then we will see what we can do together.

This level of participation of the adolescent in the discussion helps in developing the therapeutic alliance and even more allows the adolescent to exercise some form of autonomy and responsibility.

# Establishing a "Safe" Frame for the Treatment

In general, if suicidal thoughts or behavior is a manifestation of severe depression, the depression needs to be treated. If, to the contrary, it is a characterologically based suicidal intention linked to the personality disorder but not a reflection of depression, the setting up of the treatment contract with patient and family requires spelling out that the patient and, to some extent, the family, but not the therapist, are responsible for the patient's behavior outside the sessions. The patient will have to assume the contractual responsibility of either controlling his or her impulses and discussing them in the sessions or else seeking help from an emergency service of a general or a psychiatric hospital if the patient believes that he or she cannot control the suicidal impulse until the next planned session with the therapist. This difficult issue is explored in detail by Yeomans and colleagues (1992).

One important aspect of the initial diagnostic evaluation and establishment of the treatment frame is to assess to what extent the patient's pathology is supported or exacerbated to a significant degree by active family pathology, and the extent to which treatment of the family nucleus has to be part of the overall treatment arrangements. Here, again, careful assessment of the family and the patient's social environment is essential.

# Anticipating and Preventing Forms of Resistance That Could Threaten Continuation of the Treatment

Potential threats to treatment include, but are not limited to, severe self-destructive behavior with suicidal intent, and other, more indirect behavior, such as an adolescent's becoming so angry at one of his parents that he begins to doubt the continuation of treatment. Resistances can constitute patient behaviors that generate external situations that endanger the therapy.

# Beginning to Rework Maladaptive Functioning Through Behavioral Activation

It is essential for the adolescent to make the necessary efforts to become actively involved in activities of his or her age. The inactivity should be understood as an attempt to avoid the anxiety of greater emotional or relational involvement, and therefore facing anxiety by resuming activities and learning to understand its origin in terms of object relation dyads becomes a fundamental objective of the treatment.

## Agreeing to Engage With Developmental Tasks

A clear discussion must happen between the therapist and the adolescent around the objectives of the treatment. It is our understanding that the presence of a personality disorder interferes with the process of consolidation of certain psychic structures specific to adolescence, including in particular the moral and ethical system on the one hand and the integration of sexuality and aggression into the self and romantic relationships on the other hand. In addition, the process of separation-individuation that should allow greater autonomy and the development of other sources of attachment than those of parents is impacted. Our experience leads us to believe that if we do not specifically address these issues in terms of goals to be achieved, such as becoming an "honest" person or "leaving home" or "engaging in a romantic relationship," it is unlikely that the adolescent will do it on his or her own. Any delay in such a confrontation with these developmental structurations and challenges can only risk fixation of the problem and a loss of opportunity to intervene at an age when it is determined to happen.

## Establishing the Basis of Collaboration With Parents

The United States and many other countries have laws that specifically empower adolescents (14–18 years) to consent to mental health care, including psychotherapy. Parental consent is mandatory for minors under 14 years of age. However, the adolescent's right to consent to treatment does not invalidate parental authority and responsibility until the child reaches the age of majority. Therefore, parents are legally the main decision makers for their children and need to be involved in decisions that concern their well-being. They need, one way or another, to be involved in the treatment. In other words, the centrality of parents and family in the adolescent's life must be acknowledged. The parents bear legal responsibility for their child, are affected by their child's actions, and are expected by society to help shape those actions.

Also, the adolescent's impulsivity or general noncompliance may interfere with the ongoing therapy, and someone is needed (generally the parent) to facilitate or ensure the adolescent's presence at the treatment sessions. The parents may also inform the therapist about crises or significant events in the life of the adolescent or of the family that the adolescent may overlook or avoid informing the therapist about. How to accomplish these exchanges of information without violating or undermining the confidentiality agreement has to be discussed during the contracting phase.

# Case 2: William

William, a 12-year-old, hit another boy in the face because the latter touched him on the arm to indicate that he wanted his eraser back. Apparently everyone at school knows that William flies into a rage if anyone tries to touch him. The school has become increasingly concerned because this has happened a number of times, and they have threatened to expel William. They have demanded a psychiatric evaluation with the idea that William needs to be hospitalized and treated. The mother is reluctant to disclose the whole situation to the therapist because she considers that it is not William's fault, as everyone should know and respect that he does not tolerate being touched. She explains that she herself has had to accept not touching him since he was a baby, because he would cry or become angry.

It is important that a parent knows that this kind of incident needs to be communicated to the therapist so that the therapist can find a way of addressing this in the therapy and of helping William explore these difficulties.

The appropriate involvement of parents in the psychotherapy treatment may also reduce the likelihood of their sabotaging the effort. It is also valuable for the adolescent to feel the parents' support of the therapy because it will suggest that they are accepting of possible changes in the adolescent's thinking and functioning and will not suddenly withdraw the therapy if they are disappointed with the progress.

The therapist must create a confidential and private framework that facilitates the deployment of dyads of primitive object relationships in the adolescent's response to the therapist, which will be the subject of the interpretative process in TFP-A. It is common to observe deviations from planned and justified neutrality to address types of acting out that might endanger the adolescent, his or her development, or others or threaten to derail treatment. Deviations from technical neutrality are sometimes essential to protect the treatment and the patient from his or her own acting out and are inevitable when working with teenagers.

The reality principle has a link with logistical and responsibility issues: Who will bring the teenager? Who will pay for therapy? Who will inform the therapist about crises or actions that occur during the week and that may involve a threat to treatment? Who will give the key information to understand the adolescent? Because of the neurobiological features of this stage of development, adolescents are particularly at risk of acting impulsively, and this may interfere with their presence at sessions. Therefore, it is essential that someone, like a parent, can ensure that the adolescent will attend sessions or at least supervise his or her behavior.

TFP is an expensive treatment that also involves a great effort for parents, who have to organize to bring the patient twice a week and tolerate that the changes take place slowly. To protect the treatment, the therapist needs to, in the case of adolescents, also give parents some responsibilities. These responsibilities will be part of the therapeutic contract, which will be discussed later in this chapter.

Moreover, with adolescents, as noted earlier, it is necessary to communicate our understanding of the adolescent's problems and recommendation of treatment to both the adolescent and his or her parents. The therapist has to attempt to enhance the parents' understanding of the adolescent, the nature and seriousness of the child's difficulties, why TFP-A therapy is being recommended, and how it will approach the problem. We encourage parents to look for examples to understand how the pathological personality of the adolescent is the main cause of their discomfort and the difficulties they observe. In addition to talking about pathology, we help them understand and think about the consequences and likely evolution of the difficulties if there is no intervention and the adolescent does not receive help.

One concrete challenge in TFP-A is the presence of the parents in all phases of the treatment process. It introduces a complicated relationship that can be managed by agreeing on specific parameters into the treatment frame and function of the parent. The presence of parents is inevitable as well as essential. As noted earlier, parents are the main decision makers of their children, and they need, in one way or another, to be involved in the treatment. It is important to understand the pressures that parents can exert on their adolescent and the ways that they may endanger the treatment. Therefore, to protect the adolescent and the treatment, it is necessary to give the adolescent and parents some responsibilities that will inform the therapeutic contract and take into account the manner in which the pathology of the patient and parents could endanger the treatment.

# Parental Involvement in TFP-A

How does the therapist negotiate the presence of parents to ensure that the TFP-A will remain an individual treatment and that the mental activity of the therapist will primarily focus on the adolescent's internal world and the challenges of its development? Part of the answer lies in how the therapist negotiates a therapeutic contract with parents and adolescents, a process during which inevitable deviations are discussed and agreed on. The negotiation determines how the therapist will use specific tactics to protect the framework of treatment, specific techniques to return to neutrality, and specific strategies to resolve subsequent paranoid reactions to interferences, intrusions, and attacks.

First, it is important to bear in mind that parents are collaborators, not patients. This collaboration with them is structured around their real desire and parental responsibility to help the adolescent. The therapist, while acknowledging their authority, must limit their tendency to interfere or repeat traumatic experiences through the patient.

Ideally, parents should be involved as little as possible, in order to ease the normal separation process that the adolescent is gradually facing during adolescence, and only if necessary. Parental involvement is necessary when there are episodes of acting out that could harm the adolescent, his or her development, or others or threaten to derail the treatment. As we have seen, TFP-A is an individual processing in order to facilitate the deployment of the primitive object relations in the transfer. Everyone must have a shared understanding of the adolescent's problem.

Adopting a position of technical neutrality requires open and direct clarifying of the boundaries of the treatment situation and their rationale to the adolescent and his or her parents, and active, consistent educational work with the parents around the fact that they continue to maintain full authority outside of the treatment sessions. The therapist may provide recommendations regarding some problematic interactions at home, but he or she assumes no authority in this regard. The authority of the therapist is limited by the spatial boundaries of his or her office; what happens outside the office may trigger the therapist's counsel or advice, but it is not his or her responsibility.

**Parents' responsibilities.**    Parents' responsibilities must be seen as a compromise of several functions. In the first place, the parents must bring the adolescent to sessions when he or she is too young to come alone. In addition, they can remind the adolescent of the session, make it easier for the adolescent to be able to come when he or she can do it independently, and support the adolescent's participation in the therapy. If the adolescent does not want to come with the parents, they can establish a contract with him or her in which the consequences of not attending sessions are clear.

In the case of treatment in private practice, the parents should take charge of the punctual payment of the bills according to the conditions agreed with the therapist.

The adolescent is at the crossroads between childhood, aspects of which have to be abandoned, and adulthood, with the acquisition of adult skills. Ideally, the parents potentiate the adult aspects rather than the infantile aspects. However, because of the great impulsivity of this type of patient, an accompanying person is needed to guarantee the minimal conditions of the treatment. When the adolescent is reluctant to come, the parents still bring him or her. The therapist will take on the resistances of the adolescent in the transference, but it is the duty of the parents to take care of the situation and to try and bring the adolescent to the waiting room.

These are the minimum requirements. Depending on the case, it may be necessary to agree to more before initiating psychotherapy. The case of Sarah, a 14-year-old whose treatment is discussed in the next section, will illustrate how parents are involved in dealing with an adolescent's risk taking.

**Frequency of meetings with parents.**    The frequency of the therapist's meeting with the parents varies with the needs and developments in each individual case. The criteria influencing the frequency of these meetings include 1) potential dangers to the adolescent life and functioning outside the hours; 2) efforts necessary to preserve the continuity of the treatment; 3) the parents' need and requirements to receive help in managing the adolescent patient's life situation; and, most importantly, 4) the therapist's need to communicate with the parents regarding the viability of the treatment. If the treatment is not working, the parents have to be informed in the presence of the patient. It is important for the therapist, in the context of these contacts, to be concerned with protecting and respecting the autonomy of his or her patient and to be attentive to the risk that the contacts with parents, and their efforts to influence the therapist, may impact the countertransference: the therapist has to preserve his or her internal distance from the parents.

# Meeting With the Adolescent and Parents

Setting up regular joint meetings with the patient and parents—for example, every 2 months, or more frequently if the case demands it—should permit them to vent many of the problems that emerge. For example, parents may have a tendency to abandon their responsibilities, "dumping" the adolescent in the hands of the therapist; others may feel envious and resentful of the therapist's influence on their child, threatened by the therapist's potentially undermining of their authority or by the therapist's not sharing their particular ethical values and moral demands involving their child. In the case of female patients, parents may strictly forbid all sexual behavior, while the patient acts out her rebellion in unprotected sex, so that the therapist may have to help the parents find a more effective way of relating to their daughter in order to protect her from pregnancy or sexually transmitted diseases. Full discussion of all issues regarding authority in the joint meetings of adolescent, parents, and therapist should permit such a gradual clarification and assurance of the therapist's position of technical neutrality, and provide an opportunity to tease out the patient's developing transference reactions.

# Contracting

Contract setting requires agreements involving the parents, sometimes the school, and even legal authorities, in addition to those directly established with the patient. The fact that parents keep their legal authority until the adolescent reaches the age of majority gives them a certain right to be informed on a regular basis of their child's progression and the evolution of the treatment. However, the therapist has to create a space protected from the parents' intrusion where the adolescent can have the experience of autonomy and individuation. The therapist needs to systematically address all the behaviors that can put this space in jeopardy, and help to identify strategies that will protect the treatment from unnecessary intervention from the parents.

Borderline adolescents tend to evoke powerful emotional reactions in their family that influence the family's transference reactions to the therapist and heighten the influence on the treatment of the patient's transference acting out involving his or her family. These reactions may influence the parents and affect their willingness and capacity to collaborate with the treatment in terms of facilitating the adolescent's coming to sessions, being responsible regarding financial arrangements, and, especially, following through with jointly agreed-on structuring of the patient's life outside the sessions. Along these lines, parents may need help with narcissistic patients' efforts at omnipotent control, with severe acting out at home or in relation to the school. Particular difficulty may arise when the therapist has to deal with the not unusual situation in which both the parent and the adolescent strive to assert omnipotent control. Each wants to feel like the one in charge and may try to make an ally of the therapist against the other. Neither is able to let go of the other, and in this manner, each fails to facilitate greater closeness or intimacy. Further, neither easily accepts intervention from the therapist, which could threaten the maladaptive system at home.

Sometimes conflicts between the parents may be expressed in their lack of clarity regarding support for the treatment, the responsibility for the patient's attendance, and payment, and the responsibility for both of them to attend scheduled joint meetings with therapist and patient. Sometimes the suggestion may be made that parents enter into couple therapy, and in the case of separated or divorced parents, these difficulties may become even greater.

In summary, we have to find ways to integrate the parents in the treatment while bearing in mind that they generally try to do their best in these special circumstances and that no parents (or very few) want to damage their children. Optimal characteristics of parents with adolescents who would benefit from TFP-A are outlined in Table 5–1.

# Contracting With the Adolescent

Suicidal thoughts and impulses, self-harming behaviors (including serious eating disorders), drug use, and secondary benefits are considered to be threats to treatment and therefore must be incorporated into the contract. It is also necessary to establish the adolescent's responsibilities, such as the frequency of sessions (twice a week), free association, and the prioritization of the themes (i.e., when a breach in the contract occurs, the breach must be

| TABLE 5–1. | Optimal characteristics of parents with adolescents who would benefit from TFP-A |
|---|---|

Maintain scheduled appointments

Support the process

Form alliance with the psychotherapist

Limit inquiries directly to adolescent about the therapeutic process

Participate to meetings when requested

Keep psychotherapist informed about unexpected events (e.g., deaths, moves, fights)

the initial theme of the session and must be pursued until resolution is reached before discussing other themes).

The therapist must be committed to maintaining confidentiality. It is also fundamental that the therapist inform the young person about his or her availability. The therapist's responsibility is to help adolescents understand themselves so that they can make the most beneficial decisions for themselves. In further preparing the adolescent to engage in the psychotherapy, the therapist can explain that the goal is to enhance the adolescent's self-understanding, "to be able to think about yourself," although it is "natural for people to worry about what they might discover about themselves."

The contract is relatively easy to establish with adolescents who have some control over suicidality and self-harm. When this is not present, and the adolescent uses these behaviors to activate the parents, the therapist has to attempt to reduce secondary gain and evaluate whether the adolescent is ready for outpatient treatment. In these more challenging cases, the therapist may also have to introduce the idea that the behavior may hide a primitive impulse or conflict such as a desire to control or hurt the parents and the therapist.

# Case 3: Sarah

During the contracting phase with Sarah, a 14-year-old with suicidality and self-harm, the therapist observed an escalation in self-harm. For this reason, she was directed to go to the emergency room to be admitted to the psychiatric unit. It was clear that the conditions for initiating psychotherapeutic treatment were not met. She was hospitalized for 3 weeks and was discharged once the risk was reduced. Subsequently, the therapist and Sarah return to discussing the therapy contract, and Sarah agrees to try and stop self-harm and to avoid bulimic vomiting and skipping school. She agrees to talk to her parents and go to the emergency room when she feels the compulstion to harm herself. Several sessions are dedicated to discussing the contract. In order to carry out the therapy, Sarah agrees not to do any self-destructive action, including cutting, and to avoid inducements to vomiting and absences from school. If she feels the need to injure herself, she is committed to talking with her parents and going to the emergency room.

As we can see from this description, Sarah uses self-harm to split services and to capture the therapist's attention, because she seems to derive pleasure and excitement from arousing the concern of others. For example, Sarah cuts herself in the bathroom of the clinic before her session.

When the self-harm starts increasing in seriousness again, Sarah is sent to the emergency room again, but after 3 hours in the waiting room, she asks to go home. This situation is discussed with the parents, also within the framework of the contract, to help them understand that they need to insist that they need to stay until they have seen a psychiatrist in order to reduce the secondary gain without any consequences.

For the contract to help contain situations, it is essential that parents understand their child's pathology. The fact that they can understand how Sarah uses self-destructive behaviors to mobilize them and provoke a concrete response has helped them not to be influenced by their daughter's projections and to give an adequate and safe response, without giving power to the other manipulatory aspects. The fact that the parents, under the terms of the contract, brought her to the emergency room and tolerated the wait with her helped her to contain herself.

# Managing Confidentiality

An important issue in the stage of contract setting is the question of confidentiality—how patients' and family "secrets" are to be handled, as well as collateral sources of information. The general principle should be that all information regarding the patient and the sources of this information should be shared with the patient. All the material from the sessions of a therapist and an adolescent patient is confidential, with the exception of issues that the therapist considers essential to protect the patient and the treatment, which would require the therapist to contact somebody else. In the latter case, the adolescent would be told that the therapist intends to make such a contact, in order to provide the possibility of a full discussion before the therapist proceeds. It needs to be stressed that in all these cases, it is the responsibility of the therapist to indicate why such action seems essential to protect the patient's social standing, physical health, psychological well-being, or even survival. This, of course, is particularly relevant when working with adolescents who present with chronic suicidal and parasuicidal behavior, where the responsibilities of the therapist, the adolescent patient, and the family have to be clearly spelled out. On this difficult issue, we follow the recommendations of Yeomans et al. (1992) for adult patients.

# Managing Deviations From Technical Neutrality

Deviations from technical neutrality occur in order to protect adolescents from their own acting out. Since the usual aspects of support (e.g., therapeutic framework, therapist's attitude) cannot always provide enough protection for the adolescent, it is essential to introduce structural parameters to control these threats (Yeomans et al. 2015, pp. 170–171). Deviations from technical neutrality are inevitable in work with adolescents. They usually follow unsuccessful attempts by the therapist to resolve threats to treatment through clarification, confrontation, and interpretation of acting out.

For example, the therapist had to deviate from neutrality when a 19-year-old woman, Judith, wanted to leave home to live with a 50-year-old man in another state whom she had known only on the internet and with whom she had practiced cybersex. The therapist told her, "I had to insist that it was too risky to take the plane and go and stay with a man whom you had never met, and who had not come to meet your family or friends whose judgment you have always trusted. For this reason it was necessary to speak to your parents. They have the right to know and make their position clear, even though you are an adult. They did not seem to realize that they had the right to tell you that they did not want you to go, even though you are an adult. It was necessary for me to tell you about this because at that time you took an omnipotent and negligent attitude toward yourself as well as your treatment."

# Recovering From Therapist Errors and Reestablishing the Treatment Frame

As we have noted, our work with parents typically involves attempting to establish a collaborative relationship with them that allows for the development and preservation of the adolescent's individual therapy, while being careful to avoid being unwittingly drawn into a psychotherapy component with the parents. To this end, the work with parents in the TFP-A model is in service of establishing the contract and maintaining the treatment frame so that the individual psychotherapy may proceed in a productive manner. However, this may not be a simple process in which the therapist merely explains "the rules of the game." The adolescent's problems are complicated, vary in severity, and sometimes put him or her at risk, and the family/parental functioning is typically complicated as well, contributing to the development and maintenance of the adolescent's problems.

In establishing the contract, the TFP-A therapist will draw on techniques that might be considered general good practice in working with adolescents and their parents, especially within a psychodynamic framework. Yet the approach is also informed by TFP-A concepts and principles. However, when the therapist makes errors or other complications occur, other specific techniques may be utilized in order to reestablish a working space, as described in the case of Sophia.

## Case 4: Sophia

A father is concerned that the therapist broke his confidentiality by talking to his 13-year-old daughter, Sophia, about something he had told the therapist about Sophia's mother. The issue—that the mother is an active alcoholic and often uses poor judgment by engaging in activities (e.g., driving) while intoxicated that could endanger her daughter or other children—was not mentioned to the therapist by the mother or the daughter. The father tells the therapist that because of her breach, he will not talk to her anymore and will just bring his daughter to therapy. The adolescent is angry at the therapist and the father, denies that her mother has this problem, and maintains her protective stance toward the mother.

# TFP-A Principles Illustrated in the Case of Sophia

This situation incorporates many elements that highlight several principles at work in the TFP-A approach.

**Principle 1: It is important to meet with both parents/principal caretakers when taking the history and establishing the treatment contract.**    Each parent is likely to have different information that she or he believes is important to share with or shield from the therapist. As in this example, the therapist learned information from one parent about the other that was important to her role of protecting the adolescent and establishing successful treatment. Thus, problems are created when one parent hides what the other reveals. Parents also have different perspectives that broaden the therapist's understanding of the situation that the adolescent is experiencing, thereby enhancing the therapist's empathy with all parties as well as enriching the therapist's perspective on the object relations that may be established in the adolescent. One parent may try to keep the other away, either by saying the other would not be interested or by suggesting that he or she would "never come to anything," or in another situation a parent may refuse to participate.

**Principle 2: Expectations about confidentiality should be established while formulating the contract.**  Essentially, a good deal of the parenting work in TFP-A occurs early in the process. The initial work on the contract establishes and communicates the therapist's basic principle—that what is discussed with the adolescent remains confidential unless issues that threaten the safety and well-being of the adolescent, of others, or of the treatment arise. The contract states that under these conditions, the therapist will discuss with the adolescent the implementation of contract plans that involve addressing these issues with the responsible parent/caretakers to take the appropriate steps to ensure safety.

**Principle 3: The therapist must recover the treatment process when errors or other complications occur.**  In the clinical illustration, the father felt betrayed by the therapist, the adolescent was angry at father and therapist and protective of mother, and the young therapist was stunned by the adolescent's denial of the mother's alcohol problem. There remained the reality that the therapist had to confront: a) the information provided by the father indicated that the mother was in greater jeopardy than the mother or adolescent acknowledged, b) the adolescent might be in jeopardy, and c) the treatment could potentially be affected by the adolescent's denial or protection of the mother. There were several elements for the therapist to consider.

When complications occur, there are several options:

1. The therapist can acknowledge them and clarify the situation as she sees it, thereby indicating that this therapy will acknowledge and respect reality and truthfulness and will not knowingly collude with any of the participants (e.g., that the father has revealed hitherto unknown or concealed information that he does not want to have revealed to anyone

else). This process could also occur after the therapist has discussed the issue with the adolescent.

2. The therapist might request time to think about the events before deciding what to do and consult with colleagues if necessary. This option provides needed time for decision making but also serves as a model to all parties of reflection and nonimpulsive reactions that could have been pushed by emotions.

3. To regain the sense of trust and space to work in the treatment, the therapist could acknowledge that the situation might have been handled differently in a way that would not have made the parent or child feel angry, threatened, and betrayed. The concept of confidentiality could be further discussed—that the therapist had to make a decision: should she not say anything in a rigid adherence to expectations of confidentiality and "be stuck," or reaffirm that confidentiality is still wedded to the principle of protecting the child and for that purpose the parent's information was utilized as it had been? That is, the therapist may be obliged to break confidentiality to protect the parties and then work to reestablish and recover trust. A possibility like this can be discussed early in the contract formation process and then referred to later should the need arise. This approach also conveys to the participants that mistakes can be made in life, yet tolerated and resolved without irreversible harm to the situation or the individual's self-esteem. It has been our experience that more often than not, it is both accurate and useful to assume that the parent has tried to do his or her best and to convey this point of view to him or her. This point was concretely illustrated by a father who indicated, to the horror of several parents and co-therapists in a parenting group, that he hit his child with a hairbrush because he was afraid that if used his hand directly, he would be more likely to lose control and seriously hurt the child! Of course, there remain those situations where it is necessary to enlist the help of protective services to abide by legal constraints and ensure the child's safety.

**Principle 4: The therapist must be alert to identifying the relevant dyads and triads that can inform the intervention.**    In the clinical illustration, the father's hurt reaction and initial indication that he no longer would talk to the therapist suggest that he might have viewed the therapist in a somewhat idealized manner as someone who would take care of him and his daughter, unlike the way his wife did. Instead, he found a therapist who he felt acted irresponsibly. The therapist should be careful to avoid using a clinical construction like this in a manner that would subtly shift to a therapeutic mode with the father. Invocation of the reality principle might be useful:"But then I would not have your information to help her going forward" or "I'm confused. You gave me important information that was appreciated, but then you were surprised and angry that I used it. Can you see why I might have felt this way? What had you hoped I would do with this information?"

**Principle 5: The therapist must be alert to the defenses used by the parent and have an awareness of the dynamics of the situation to be in control of the countertransference.**  The therapist is alert to the father's use of splitting, his wish to force his daughter away from the mother, his insensitivity to his daughter's feelings, and his attempt to make the therapist his ally only (followed by anger and disappointment). The father is also injured in that neither the therapist nor protective services saw him as he wished to be seen, as the good parent who should have sole custody of the child. Recognizing that she is feeling the same pulls as the adolescent to take sides with one parent against the other, the therapist works to reestablish boundaries and reaffirm the father's role to get his daughter to therapy. The therapist might acknowledge the father's disappointment with her ("I realize I have disappointed you") but reaffirm that all of the parties, in their own unique way in their role in the adolescent's life, are working to help her be safe, improve, and grow.

# Understanding Challenges for Adolescents Who Have Experienced Abuse or Neglect

## Case 5: Catherine

Catherine, a 13-year-old, is referred by a child abuse protection agency after having been sexually abused (i.e., fondling, sexual touching) by her mother's previous boyfriend. Her mother has a long history of severe alcoholism and violence, especially toward Catherine's father, which led to their divorce, as well as toward her frequently changing boyfriends. Child custody has been contentious since the divorce. Catherine has no friends and is bullied at school because of her slight overweight appearance. She has scars on her forearms but denies self-mutilation, and mentions having anxiety and depressive thoughts.

She is happy to meet a therapist, saying that she prefers to be with adults than with friends her age. She looks neglected in her clothing and is quite talkative, but the content of her speech is very superficial (e.g., talks about tricks that her dog does, visits that she makes to the shopping mall with her mom, TV shows that she watches when at her dad's). When asked to specify her difficulties, she indicates problems at school and not liking anyone because everyone is "mean and stupid." She makes no mention of the sexual abuse and the family problems. A few sessions later, when confronted with her mother's alcohol problems, her possibly witnessing violence at home, and her facing the anguish of possibly losing her mother, who was pursued by the justice system after being arrested for drunk driving, Catherine denies everything, becomes verbally aggressive toward the therapist, and immediately discloses the content of the session to her mother, who becomes furious and asks for a change in therapists.

It is our experience that many children and adolescents, especially those who have experienced chronic abuse, emotional deprivation, or parental antipathy, face common issues, including:

1. Feeling a perverse "loyalty" toward the parents who abused and neglected them. They behave as if they have an obligation to protect the parents from being exposed by the rest of the world. In our illustration, Catherine was able to collaborate because she was not threatened by the therapist, who tolerated her triviality for a while. However, had the therapist reacted differently and not correctly understood Catherine's actions as an attempt to protect herself from a deeper conflict, it could have created a situation in which the adolescent would have been perceived as deliberately hiding information or lying to the therapist.
2. Blaming themselves for the abuse or neglect because they believed that deep down they were "bad children," not because they had "bad parents," which for survival purposes would be a disastrous thought. This would mean that they were always in danger and could die at any time. At least, by thinking that they are responsible, they can believe they retain a certain power to influence their parents, by protecting them, but at the cost of neglecting their needs for those of their parents. Fairbairn (1952) called this the "moral defense." Using the moral defense, they mislead themselves into thinking that if they were not so "bad," the abuse would stop and the "bad parent" would become the "good parent."
3. Maintaining the fantasy that they had some control over a situation in which they were truly helpless.
4. Staying attached to the internal bad object in such a way that they avoid or reject acceptance, understanding, and friendship and prefer uncaring, neglecting, and abusive ones. For example, Catherine had no friends, stayed at home most of the time, and refused to come to treat-

ment as soon as she was confronted with the reality of an unprotective family environment. It may be appropriate and useful to consider that the bullying condition at school, which she did not really complain about, helps her to maintain that fragile equilibrium between "being helpless" and "being in control" or between "her mom being bad" and "the rest of the world being mean."

5. Being suspicious of the motives of potentially helpful others. If these adolescents ever gain the capacity to tolerate a more realistic view of their parents or they take the risk to trust someone without the fantasized or real fear of retaliation from the parents, they will always have to face another challenge—namely, their suspiciousness of the motives of potentially helpful others, expecting that at any moment these "good objects" could turn "bad" and become abusive like the parents were. In addition, the suspiciousness could include a disbelief that anyone would want good things for them and, in the face of that possibility, not feel afraid that others' envy would seek to deprive them or retaliate for the good experience.

All these themes will have to be dealt with within the transference.

# Reviewing the Contract and Recontracting

In this chapter, we specified the first tactic in TFP-A, which is the establishment of an initial treatment contract with the adolescent and his or her parents to address urgent difficulties that may threaten the adolescent's physical integrity or survival and that of other people, and conditions that will guarantee the continuation of the treatment. After covering the usual arrangements of a psychodynamic treatment, the contract specifies conditions under which the treatment can be carried out that involve certain responsibilities and power for the adolescent and certain responsibilities for the parent and the therapist. What is also important is to eliminate the secondary gain of the behavior and ensure a minimum of collaboration of both adolescent and parents. It is also important in these contract arrangements at the beginning of the treatment that the therapeutic structure eliminate the secondary gain of treatment and ensure a minimum of collaboration with the parent.

A variety of factors may impel the therapist to seek *recontracting*. As the treatment proceeds, the therapist may hear about problems that already existed but were previously not expressed by the patient, or known problems may worsen, requiring therapist and patient to amend the contract. For example, an awareness or new appearance of, say, eating problems or drug use may require the therapist to initiate discussion about a modification of the treatment contract, including incorporating an outside treatment intervention to address these problems.

A change in the patient's life circumstance will require all therapists, not just TFP-A therapists, to modify the contract and reexamine treatment goals. For example, should the family change living arrangements in a manner that affects the viability of the treatment, the plan will have to be converted to a time-limited intervention. The TFP-A therapist, in discussion with adolescent and parents, may have to consider a triage approach and identify which goals to focus on and which to give less attention to while acknowledging with the adolescent that this change is one they have little control over. To not do this would be equivalent to the therapist joining the adolescent or the parents in denying that this change is having an impact and is being forced on them. That could contribute to further frustration, reduce the likelihood of any positive gains from the therapy that could still take place, and make the patient more hesitant about resuming therapy at a later time or with a new therapist when circumstances allow.

This change may affect also the therapist's decisions about the utilization of TFP techniques. For example, some may decide to avoid transference interpretation if they feel this will open lines of thinking and experiences of affect that cannot be resolved because of insufficient time available to reach a resolution. An alternative, chosen by some therapists, is to offer deep, very integrative interpretations so that the adolescent is given a perspective that he or she will be highly likely to reflect on and consider outside the session. This would also be something the adolescent could explore if he or she will be entering another therapy. This approach is derived from the TFP concept of offering the patient this type of interpretation when the therapy is in jeopardy and the patient appears to be set to leave against advice, indicating that the therapist's other comments have not been truly heard or thought about. This type of an interpretation would try to incorporate the therapist's understanding of the patient's refusal or inability to judge the situation in a more adaptive and constructive manner. In the type of situation discussed here, it could include a comment on the adolescent's feeling that he or she is being adversely affected by parental decisions that have invalidated and not taken into consideration his or her wishes or needs, resulting in acting out in a way that is maladaptive and possibly harmful.

# CHAPTER 6

# Techniques of TFP-A

**TREATMENT TECHNIQUES** essentially refer to the therapist's methods of communicating therapeutically and addressing what happens in the here and now of the session and moment to moment between the therapist and the adolescent. They include the establishment of a "holding environment," an active stance of the therapist, the interpretative process, transference and countertransference analysis, and technical neutrality. Although these key techniques of Transference-Focused Psychotherapy for Adolescents (TFP-A) have been adapted from the techniques used in Transference-Focused Psychotherapy (TFP) with adults, there are important technical differences that help the therapist respond optimally to the needs specific to working with adolescents, especially adolescents with borderline personality disorder (BPD). Two of the most notable differences in TFP-A are the much more active stance of the therapist and the importance of clarification.

The treatment techniques we describe are methods that the therapist uses to communicate with the adolescent, with the goal of increasing the adolescent's self-reflection and awareness, generating curiosity and a better understanding of his or her inner experiences, and promoting development toward greater identity consolidation and change in problematic functioning. They include the statements directed toward the adolescent as well as those techniques that inform and guide the therapist about which techniques to deploy and how and when to use them. They form the basis of the moment-to-moment interactions between therapist and adolescent that call attention to what is happening in the here and now of the session. Essentially, they are the procedures that are thought to have a therapeutic impact—that promote the desired change in adolescent personality organization and behavioral expression.

The impact of the developmental differences on technique is reflected in two technical features, in particular, that the TFP-A therapist keeps in mind to optimize work with adolescents. First, the therapist must adopt and maintain a much more active stance with adolescents. Second, the therapist must deploy techniques of the interpretative process differently with adolescents. For example, the procedures of clarification and confrontation build toward setting the stage for interpretation proper, but with adolescents, clarification may take on greater import than with adults.

The developmental status and demands of adolescents are distinct from those of adults and younger children. As the adolescent grows through this phase, he or she has to make progress on the work of establishing an identity that intersects with a movement toward a sense of autonomy, a further-developing sense of separateness and internal differentiation, while succumbing neither to a pull to regress nor to a sadness or fear about being less dependent. Therefore, the confident and effective use of these techniques in the work with adolescents requires a particular awareness and sensitivity on the part of the therapist to create a setting—a *holding environment,* so to speak (Winnicott 1962/1965; 1971)—that fosters the conditions that make the adolescent feel safe despite these typically unconscious developmental demands as well as the conflicts that emanate from his or her personality disorder and from being in an exploratory psychotherapy.

# Holding Environment

As in any psychotherapeutic milieu, the TFP-A therapist needs to create a setting in which the adolescent and the therapist can explore and express thoughts and feelings. Because TFP-A asks the patient to free associate, the patient needs to feel that he or she can say whatever comes to mind without feeling fear of criticism, humiliation, rejection, or abandonment. Furthermore, because TFP-A places an emphasis on the therapist's sensitivity toward and awareness of the ongoing affect in the session, both adolescent and therapist must feel safe with its expression so that it can be utilized as conceived in the treatment model. This requires that the therapist be able to comment on the expressed affect of the moment without promoting avoidance or dissociation, while also being able to offer an interpretation that will broaden understanding of the experience.

The creation of such an environment requires an alertness to the adolescent's attachment style and its impact on how she experiences the separation-individuation process and moves toward autonomy and independence. Because predominant affects that can come into play in these situations are anxiety and aggression, the therapist faces the challenge of being sensitive to the anxiety without becoming supportive in a way that could engender secondary gains derived from the adolescent's helplessness or create a regressive condition that would promote the adolescent's need to flee. The aggression expressed by the adolescent in sessions can often be accompanied by a paranoid quality and projective elements. This can put the therapist at risk of engaging in an enactment of the battles the adolescent may be having with her parents if the therapist experiences a countertransference that induces the adolescent to try to impose strict or inappropriate limits. Alternatively, the therapist, like the parents, may feel like he is "walking on eggshells" and become constricted and not be able to describe, confront, or set limits when he is afraid of an aggressive reaction by the adolescent.

This early phase of the work can have as one of its goals to begin creating a setting that clearly values promoting the adolescent's capacity to reflect on himself and, by doing so, begin to have a different reaction when he experiences affect, for example, an alternative to freezing, avoidance, fleeing, anger, or even dissociation—something other than fight or flight.

Many qualities contribute to creating this environment, especially the therapist's warmth, empathy, and understanding, long-recognized therapist features that help make any therapeutic approach successful. In addition, the TFP-A therapist may utilize scaffolding at various times, perhaps more so in the early part of the treatment, that helps the patient learn how to engage in TFP-A. This scaffolding involves taking small steps that create conditions that allow for interventions such as confrontation and, later, interpretation. It is not just an issue of timing. It involves a recognition that the therapist can gradually address the deficits that contribute to the adolescent's borderline personality organization (BPO), sometimes through support or psychoeducation, while building toward the opportunity to offer an interpretation that can have significant impact.

At the same time, the therapist must be aware of the possibility that the holding environment may evoke even more anxiety and, often, suspiciousness in the adolescent, such that she may either look like she is collaborating, rapidly agreeing with the therapist but lying and hiding important matters, or become openly and aggressively rejecting, mute, or actively contemptuous. It is not unusual to adopt a balanced strategy between involving the parents and suggesting a deep interpretation of that reaction in an understanding way and offering a confrontation on the way the adolescent is stuck. (For example, on the one hand, she may want to be autonomous and free, but on the other hand, she behaves or uses means [e.g., drugs] in such a way to worry and involve others.)

A procedure such as this may occur during the course of one session or across sessions. For example, Anna, the 19-year-old whose case was discussed in Chapter 4, in a family session said that she could not tolerate and certainly not talk about the upset she was feeling when she and her parents brought up how awful they all felt and still feel when they think about her being sent away to a residential program. She threatened that she would leave the session if the therapist decided to persist with this topic. The therapist provided an empathic comment and stated that this issue would not be pursued at this time. He asked if he could explain why he thought that being able to talk about such feelings at some point would be a therapeutic goal so that she would have other options besides avoidance of her inner life or threatening to flee others. She agreed, and the therapist explained. It was felt that this supportive intervention paved the way for a point later in the session when Anna accepted and worked with an interpretation that her inconsistent presence at home and the manner in which fights occurred, followed by her storming out for days, reflected her attempt at mastery over being sent away, but that now, in a role reversal, she is the one in charge of leaving, and her parents are the ones who are helpless to stop it and are terrified, not knowing when she would return and if she was safe. Other illustrations of this concept are provided in this chapter that illustrate the joint deployment of supportive and interpretative techniques.

# Active Stance of the Therapist

In working with adolescents, especially adolescents with BPD, the stance of the therapist is somewhat different from the stance therapists generally assume with adult patients. The active stance we propose the therapist assume was evident in the approach displayed by Paulina Kernberg in videos of her work. Although most who are trained as child and adolescent therapists may take this for granted, they may differ significantly in what they consider to be the appropriate level of therapist activity. In the active stance, the therapist adopts a neutral, nonjudgmental position yet shows expressive facial reactions and actively communicates a warm and friendly interest in the adolescent and his or her experiences. The activity is best reflected in the therapist's being engaged and avoiding long periods of silence while showing interest and enthusiasm or being playful or instructive when necessary. Qualities such as these are illustrated in the case of the high school boy (mid-BPO) who told his therapist that he told a joke in class and got into trouble. "You want to hear it?" he asked. The therapist said yes and was told that during a class discussion of the Great Depression, the patient had commented that they could also study the "great depression" at their school because there was so much of it. Thus, the therapist joined the boy in an experience of which he seemed somewhat proud and could expand discussion of that experience by commenting that the boy was right—that although this was inappropriate for that particular classroom and the therapist could understand the teacher's reaction, the therapist could acknowledge that it was funny and especially that the humor was meaningful and, in fact, poignant. This comment could then lead into their discussion of depression the boy might be feeling. This kind of interchange conveys to the patient a flexibility and openness by the therapist and a comfort with the boy's affect.

TFP-A therapists are always alert to providing comments that stimulate thought and responses from the adolescent. To do this, therapists must remain alert to countertransference, not only to avoid their own acting out but also to provide a model, though unexpressed, of persons who can focus on their internal state, reflect on their affect to enhance self-understanding, and inform their comments as they heighten their awareness of the affectively dominant object relation active at that moment.

The purpose of adopting such a benign, warm, and active stance is derived from the interpersonal qualities and history often seen in adolescents who show BPO and from the nature of the BPO psychopathology itself. First, for the adult therapist to be seen as someone who has value to the adolescent, active engagement may be especially important with these youngsters, who have not consistently experienced the benign interest of adults. So the objective is to communicate such an interest and to create a therapeutic safe space where the adolescent feels free to begin to express and explore his or her reactions and thoughts. It is of great value to facilitate engagement and communication with adolescents because they may be inclined to try and sort out their difficulties on their own or to confide in others of their age. Interacting in this way should clearly be distinct from becoming friendly or a friend, which many parents and adolescents consider to be an essential characteristic in selecting a therapist, as in the case of one parent who supported her daughter's preference to see a particular male therapist who was "cool and wore an earring." Second, because research shows that adolescents with BPO often interpret neutral faces as malevolent (Scott et al. 2011), therapists who insist on or tend to maintain a "blank screen" facial expression may hinder engaging the adolescent in treatment and provoke the paranoid perspective that many BPO adolescents can bring to a session. This unnecessarily interferes with establishing a relationship of trust by which it is possible to express and explore concerns and to begin the work of mutually elaborating understanding that will be central for stabilizing and integrating affect and consolidating identity.

Being active also helps the therapist keep the focus on what is happening in the session and makes it less likely for the adolescent, either consciously or without awareness, to shift her commentary to outside details that can sometimes be less important and distracting. Of course, an up-to-date awareness of outside events (e.g., school, family, friendships, relationships, and especially features related to the frame) is welcomed by the therapist. The active engagement enhances the likelihood of identifying relevant dyads and transferential elements. Thus, the transference develops despite this active stance, which does not interfere with the development and exploration of dyads and affects that have to be addressed, clarified, and interpreted in TFP-A.

The active stance and the elements that promote it are important for getting the process of communication going and to sustain it and gradually help the adolescent to develop the capacity to express what is on her mind and move toward free association when possible. Before free association is possible, the therapist needs to use clarification, providing scaffolding for the thinking and communication process through probes, comments, and restatements that feed the adolescent's sense of agency in elaborating narratives, putting her experience into words, and sharing and elaborating this with the therapist. The therapist may also utilize supportive techniques to help move the process toward free association and interpretative goals.

The therapist may also turn to these techniques of being active and in the moment when it is necessary to work with the family. Here, too, the clinician must be alert to verbal, nonverbal, affective, and countertransferential modes of communication. By maintaining simultaneous awareness to what is said, to actions that accompany speech and silence, and to the guiding role that the impact of these verbal and nonverbal behaviors can have on him or her, the clinician can maintain a focus on moment-to-moment transactions, the here and now of the therapy session, and interactions of the moment. In the example earlier, with Anna, the therapist's understanding and identification of the fight-separation-reunion sequence they experienced, which was now a looming threat in the session, and its subsequent interpretation, came about as a result of the therapist being very active and immediately picking up on a snappiness that suddenly happened between mother and daughter. The daughter was unnecessarily provoked by the mother and responded almost "on cue." Then, the therapist integrated this moment with relevant history and missed therapy sessions. Still later, it was noted that the mother's negative comments led Anna to take on the role of the "bad" one, which was then enacted in arenas such as her employment difficulties—her worry that her boss would find her to be incompetent/bad/stupid and would get rid of her. By not working, she avoided the shame of feeling inadequate and disappointing to herself.

# Illustration of TFP-A Techniques

The clinical example that follows offers commentary on a few features from a single psychotherapy session to illustrate how the TFP-A approach might sound. It introduces fundamental TFP-A techniques that include clarification, confrontation, and the use of countertransference and interpretation while maintaining technical neutrality. After familiarizing the reader with the deployment of concepts in this session, we then offer more comprehensive explanations of these TFP-A techniques and provide additional clinical examples that elaborate on the techniques.

## Case 1: Claire

Claire, a 17-year-old high school student, was bright and hoped to do well at school and to attend university but did not give her schoolwork the devotion required to readily achieve her goals. She was sexually promiscuous and abused alcohol, elements that were incorporated into the frame and required "recontracting" when it became clear that she continued to engage in risky behaviors that were dangerous to her. For example, her sexual promiscuity left her vulnerable to sexually transmitted disease and to exploitation by young men, and there was a concern that she had become pregnant. She came to recognize that her alcohol use led her to behave in ways she might feel shame about when sober, and an alcohol prevention intervention was being considered, in a recontracting, that would be separate from her TFP-A psychotherapy. She could express the realization that her drinking was harmful and self-destructive, but with regard to following through on this awareness and limiting her drinking, she said she would ignore it: "I don't care about it." Despite this, Claire maintained an investment in her psychotherapy and attended in a regular and timely manner and developed a connection to her female psychotherapist. As psychotherapy proceeded, Claire showed a greater level of self-awareness and expressed dismay that if she could view herself while drunk, dancing, and acting in a sexually overt manner, she would feel shame. She recognized the disparity between how she behaved and the behavior that would have reflected her more idealized self representation.

In one session Claire described her concern, which she expressed to her boyfriend, that he was just seeing her to "have sex" and had no deeper feeling for her. She told him she wanted to see him "but not just for that." He was upset that she thought he felt that way toward her. She seemed uncertain whether she could believe his protest; told her therapist, "I don't give a damn"; and then suddenly expressed regret that she no longer saw her father. She said that her father had barely acknowledged her birthday, which had just occurred, that he hardly knew anything about her life now, and that she longed to see him regularly, because "when I see him I'm fine." Her parents are divorced, and Claire has a long history of being neglected, albeit in a different manner, by each of them. After expressing this regret about not seeing her father, Claire said, "Well, it doesn't matter, it's okay."

How might a therapist approach these comments by this adolescent? One way might be to take an empathic stance and to comment, "You sound sad and angry toward these men in your life" and even note that after stating her feelings she then dismisses them, as though they are unimportant. Such a comment would represent an attempt to label the affect and to draw Claire out, to have her be more in touch with her feelings and perhaps have a greater awareness of her internal experiences, consider their impact, and not be so quick to dismiss or minimize them. There is value in this.

The TFP-A perspective also considers affect to be important and tries to identify the dominant affect in the session. However, in the TFP-A model we do not just name the affect or consider affect in isolation, but always clarify affect as part of a dyad of self-other representations. For example, rather than telling a patient, "You seem angry about that" (referring to something the patient believed the therapist did or thought), the TFP-A therapist might offer, "So, it's as if I'm mean and don't seem to care very much about you, and you are trapped and have to come here and suffer or your parents will get even angrier at you." In this case, the transference is utilized to elaborate on the object relations dyad and associated affect in a clarifying statement provided by the therapist. In doing this, the focus moves from solely commenting on something "internal" to the patient to offering a description with a more externalized quality to the dyad that can be jointly examined and discussed.

With regard to Claire, the TFP-A therapist might have offered a comment such as, "So, with both your father and your boyfriend you seem to see yourself as expendable, to be available when it is convenient to them, but then you dismiss or blow off your anger, as though you don't believe it's safe or justified for you to allow yourself to have such a feeling, perhaps worrying that they would abandon you altogether." Then, depending on Claire's thoughts about this observation, the therapist might have added a comment about her defensive style: "Indeed, you then often blame yourself, such as when you said maybe it would be different if you had written more to your father." In effect, the therapist is developing an idea with Claire that can be explored and expanded on as they discuss other examples—namely, that she sees herself as "the bad one," with her father's treatment of her as consistent with this self representation. This allows her to take on blame and continue to play out this role in daily life outside the classroom (e.g., be exploited sexually by others) while unconsciously maintaining an idealized representation of her father. This self-conceptualization gets extended such that her boyfriend, who seems to care for her, gets portrayed as someone who superficially cares for her and uses her as needed. This reaction seems to occur when the sadness, driven by feeling neglected, gets activated.

The TFP-A therapist might also utilize clarification and ask Claire to talk more about her feeling of "not caring." Confrontation would also be integrated into the discussion ("I'm struck by something and wondered what you thought. You describe feeling upset, angry, and ashamed and express a sense of being neglected and exploited—strong feelings!—and then you say things like 'who cares' or 'it's all right.' What do you make of that?"). Similarly, when Claire describes the "horrible" moments when she is drunk and can hardly stand, but likes it, she can be asked to clarify, to tell more about that experience that makes her like it so much. She had described that when she was so drunk, even nauseous, the feeling was "beautiful" because "I'm not afraid of anything." Claire had been discussing her discomfort in feeling anger or sadness because she felt helpless to do anything about it, and so the therapist might use confrontation to ask her to reflect on her sense of helplessness and impotence when she is sober and feeling sad and the omnipotence she experiences when she is drunk, numb, and disconnected from her internal world and even from her friends' opinion of her at that moment. This reversal of how she experiences herself when drunk (impotence to omnipotence) relieves her from concern about shame and being the bad, unwanted, neglected one. In summary, the therapist, while attentive to the affect, also tries to integrate it with the adolescent's self and other representations and to examine defenses and changes in affect and object representations.

This theme of Claire's feelings of impotence and her use of omnipotence can be further studied by examining it with regard to her interactions with the therapist in the transference. For example, when Claire provides illustrations and states how "bad" she is and how helpless or unmotivated she feels to change herself, she leaves the therapist in a helpless, frustrated state. Although Claire also seems to be helpless, she may find significant secondary gain in the sympathy she receives from some people, including at times the therapist, for the awful life position in which she finds herself. However, she is also quite omnipotent, controlling sessions by repeating stories reflecting the danger she creates for herself and the maladaptive or ineffective approach she takes toward trying to grow up. While stuck, such an adolescent can become powerful and make the therapy feel frozen as well.

Claire's treatment situation illustrates how adolescents may distance themselves from their anxiety and how, because they may have little motivation to change, techniques like confrontation can be used to "rock the boat" and move them toward owning a level of anxiety they can contain. To this point, Claire can maintain a status quo by seeing herself as "the bad one" or occasionally blaming a parent or friend. The TFP-A techniques hope to move the adolescent toward a greater awareness of her concern about herself, and the use of the transference relation can play an important role here. Most importantly, comments such as those described here might be the sort that would help Claire reflect on her behavior and move her toward examining and reaffirming the frame. Utilizing TFP-A techniques may also offer the therapist a level of awareness and tools to forestall being drawn in, either by countertransference pressures or a rigid adherence to rules, and taking on the role of being the strict parent (that Claire never had).

Claire's dangerous behaviors may be viewed as an acting out of the representations of split self/other dyads (e.g., the good girl who wants to do well in school, feel proud, and make her parents proud, and the bad girl who cannot control impulses, feels shame when realizing how others may see her, and feels sadness about being maltreated but actually feels omnipotent because she obliterates her anxiety and feels all-powerful or invincible at such a moment). If the representations that support this acting out can be brought into the transference, brought "inside" the session, it may help contain the acting-out behaviors that occur "outside" and eventually help serve as the medium of change that fosters growth in the adolescent's reflective functioning, awareness of self, and integration of split representations. The transference, reminiscent of the child's use of a transitional object, may serve as a safe space where the affect and the associated self/other associations may be "played out." For this to successfully occur, the therapist must maintain technical neutrality so that the adolescent can come to recognize that the affect is hers, to become internalized and contained. For example, in working in the transference, it may be possible for the therapist to put into words something that Claire cannot do or avoids doing—expressing the reality that her father is neglecting her—and explain that if Claire continues to act out and flaunt to the therapist how reckless she is, and get away with it without limit setting, then she also converts the therapist into a neglecting object. By drawing Claire's attention to the self-neglect expressed through her acting out, she may come to realize her identification with the neglecting object and to understand how the adolescent males she selects will repeatedly re-create that dyad of a neglecting object and a neglected self. As she continues, unconsciously, to seek the idealized father she wishes for, she escapes having awareness of how neglected she has been and continues to be. When her boyfriend tried to express loving feelings toward her, she minimized and ridiculed them, in a sense turning the tables on him and becoming the distant one while maintaining her status of neglect.

It is our belief that the interpretation of elements like these, which is also helped by the use of clarification and confrontation, contributes to helping the adolescent move from a position of stasis toward the inherent growth trajectory of adolescent identity formation, more developmentally appropriate self-awareness, and a direction of maturity involving separation and autonomy. All of this is approached by framing comments that still maintain attention to the adolescent's internal experiences while trying to reflect a degree of distance from that internal world so the adolescent may join in examining it rather than defending or running from it.

# Interpretative Process

The therapist is active and engaged with adolescents, and several of the TFP techniques that were developed for adults (Caligor et al. 2007; Yeomans et al. 2015) can be deployed with adolescents, but sometimes with adaptations. The therapist needs to be alert to verbal, nonverbal, affective, and countertransferential modes of communication. As noted earlier, by maintaining simultaneous awareness to what is said, to actions that accompany speech and silence, and to the guiding role that the impact of these verbal and non-verbal behaviors can have, the therapist can maintain a focus on moment-to-moment transactions. By focusing on the here and now of the therapy session—the interaction of the moment—the therapist pays attention to qualities of the adolescents' cognitive construction and verbal expression that may be characteristic in many situations, especially those that have the emotional demands that are found in many social interactions.

When thinking about the techniques of TFP-A, the cognitive demands of the therapy interaction and features of the cognitive development of adolescence should be considered jointly because they, along with the conclusions about the severity of psychopathology that arose in the assessment, inform qualities of the therapist's intervention. The therapist's comments are neither declarative or directly concrete (e.g., "You are…") nor invasive (e.g., "You are thinking/feeling that…") but descriptive (e.g., "It seems that you are acting as though…"; "Could it be that you feel as though no one wants to give you anything, like a rejected, ignored child might feel…?")

and have the quality of a metaphor whose understanding, in some form, continues to develop through adolescence into young adulthood, in part influenced by the continuing development of executive functioning (Carriedo et al. 2016). The "as though" construction in the therapist's comment requires that the patient be able to move beyond the concrete, to not be constrained by how things look. Elkind (1967) pointed out that the school-age child may not be able to distinguish between hypotheses, mental creations, and actual perceptual data, but the adolescent can. The adolescent develops the ability to think and reason about his own thought and the thoughts of others. He can think of all possible combinations in a problem, indicating that he can imagine and reason about what might be and not only what is. Therefore, he can step back from the moment and consider an "as though" statement as though it were true, reason about it, and consider that things could be different from how they are (Elkind 1967).

However, Elkind (1967) pointed out a form of egocentrism that is a negative by-product of each new stage of cognitive development, as described by Piaget, and that diminishes during the development of that period. For the adolescent, the egocentrism is reflected in the construction of a "collective audience" and a "personal fable." Although adolescence brings with it the ability to "think about thinking," adolescents may, at the beginning, think that others are thinking about what they are thinking about—namely, themselves. This collective audience diminishes by 15 or 16 years of age, prompted by interactions with others. It can feel to the therapist that this feature is in operation with those adolescents who seem to expect that the therapist will automatically and magically understand them, regardless of what they say or how they say it. The personal fable arises from the egocentric feature of feeling unique and special and may diminish because of involvement in more intimate relations.

A feature of adolescent cognitive growth that may be especially valuable to recognize is the continuing development of processing capacity from early childhood to early adolescence that allows for a greater number of dimensions to be simultaneously represented (Case and Okamoto 1996; Halford and Andrews 2006; Kuhn and Franklin 2006). The adolescent's developing competence with understanding structural complexity, growth in working memory and executive functioning, and movement from the concrete to the abstract provides the potential to process and work with the TFP-A therapist's comments, which are intended to promote personality integration by working with the defenses that have been interfering with this growth. This allows the therapist to verbalize the various contradictions that typically exist in the thinking of individuals with BPD and to present before them, simultaneously, these features (perhaps presented as dyads), which are typically dissociated in these individuals, but which they, as adolescents, now have the cognitive capacity to become aware of because of their ability to focus on several features at one time. Over time, this process makes it harder for an adolescent (or adult) to maintain these contradictions as separate constructions experienced in an ego-syntonic manner.

# Clarification

Things should make sense, so when a patient's comments are vague, when causal links are not clear or absent, or when gaps in the narrative arise, *clarification* may be used to see if the adolescent can understand why the other person might be confused and whether she can provide a clearer, better organized response. Clarification is a central TFP-A technique because so many adolescents do not yet have the ease and facility to think about, express, and communicate their affective experience and concerns. Clarification is often used with adolescents (and adults), especially while they are gaining experience as therapy participants and learning to recognize that a certain degree of clarity and specificity in their commentary is necessary for them to be truly understood by the therapist. The therapist asking for clarification reflects that the collective audience is not operative—that the therapist does not know what the adolescent meant unless it is expressed with clarity—and drives the realization that the therapist is separate, with independent thoughts and understanding. Thus, the therapist plays an active role in helping and keeping the clarification going until the adolescent develops the capacity to do this with less and less scaffolding from the therapist. We have shown previously in a number of empirical studies that children, adolescents, and adults with mental health problems, including BPD, as well as those who have experienced abuse and neglect, frequently have a very limited sense of themselves and others and generally are inclined to focus only on the behavioral rather than the psychological. In work with such patients, some scaffolding helps to get this ability going.

The therapist may continue to need to ask for clarification on an issue until the adolescent's vagueness becomes minimal and, in so doing, helps the adolescent recognize the inconsistencies and contradictions in his thinking (Caligor et al. 2018). The therapist can use clarification in a disarming way so that the adolescent does not feel assaulted by a series of questions that makes him feel inadequate. For example, the therapist could take the onus of (mis)understanding from the adolescent and say, "I wasn't sure if I understood. Could you tell me more about that?" or "Let me check if I understood correctly.

Could you say more about…" or "Let me see if I've got this right…" The therapist repeats her understanding of the adolescent, who can then correct her if necessary. With regard to lapses in explaining causal sequences, the therapist might say, "I understood what you said about 'a' and about 'b' and 'c,' but could you explain more how you got from 'a' to 'c'?" These approaches may be needed more frequently with younger adolescents.

Because clarification is a technique that is utilized for all ages, its use is not solely prompted by cognitive developmental limitations, and its requirement suggests that the adolescent is expressing something about an area of conflict and that a defense is operative. Clarification is much more likely to be needed when splitting defenses are in play, because they are associated with more vague or partial responses that can be difficult for the therapist to follow. Patients at a more severe BPO level may become more frustrated, angrier, and more confused when the therapist expresses confusion over the patient's vague replies. If the adolescent feels more frustrated and foolish, she can react with anger, as if she believes the therapist is trying to "make her look bad." However, if she can be helped to appreciate that this whole sequence is occurring because the therapist very much wants to understand her and not be mistaken or misrepresent what the adolescent is thinking and feeling, this repeated process may lead the adolescent to become more aware of and more clearly express her inner and external experience. In a subtle way it leads to more reflection and a realization that words, more so than actions, can effectively express her experiences.

For some adolescents, an ongoing need for clarification may reflect a hostile resistance, perhaps on a continuum with those who remain silent and refuse to talk. The adolescent may also be inviting the therapist to act in a way that is experienced as critical, enacting a dyad in which the adolescent is the disliked child who can never say or do anything that pleases or satisfies the parent. The countertransference can inform the therapist if this is an avenue that might be pursued. Other adolescents may be vague because they are afraid of being known or understood, perhaps because they are trying to protect a family secret. Their confusion can indicate the need for confrontation.

# Confrontation

Confrontation is utilized in the presence of contradictions (verbal and nonverbal), omissions, and inconsistencies in the adolescent's narrative. This is not a hostile, judgmental intervention; rather, it is a supportive attempt that points out to the adolescent the things she is saying that reflect contradictory internal states that might not make sense to a listener. It can then be observed if the adolescent can reflect on the interviewer's comment, understand why the response seemed confusing or inconsistent, and show flexibility and reorganize her thoughts and present them in a coherent manner rather than in the more chaotic manner she first used.

Confrontation becomes a very important technique, particularly in the early stages of treatment. Confrontation can be used to draw attention to the patient's behavior in the sessions and to invite the patient to think about and consider whatever drew the attention of the therapist. This is likely to play an essential role in helping the adolescent become aware of affects such as anger and rage or affective and defensive reactions, for example, retreating to a haughty, dismissive superiority when he feels hurt or misunderstand, that he would otherwise not have the opportunity to see within himself. These are all important roads to exploring transference dispositions evident in the nonverbal reactions of adolescents with BPD and powerful affects and self/ other representations of which he may be quite unaware. In this way, the therapist's capacity to confront and find a way to talk about and bring into awareness the elephant in the room, to describe and talk in a matter-of-fact way about what may be uncomfortable, and to help the adolescent think about it may add a great deal of value in bringing into awareness something that may be a key part of the puzzle regarding his reactions and the reactions of others to him.

Confrontations lead, however, not necessarily to immediate transference interpretation but rather to the relationship of what evolves in the session to the patient's behaviors outside the session, thus facilitating the analysis of transference dispositions expressed toward third parties before direct interpretation of the transference. Confrontation may also become an important technique in cases in which the adolescent receives significant secondary gain (e.g., using her "psychiatric illness" to justify her absence from classes and exams) that may have to be vigorously confronted and resolved in order for it not to become a major obstacle to progress in the treatment and to the adolescent's development and engagement with phase-appropriate developmental tasks. Here, the therapist may have to explore and engage the adolescent with thinking about the consequences of not doing her homework, smoking pot in places where she is likely to be caught, or engaging in risky sexual behavior so that they can work out what can be done to minimize the risk of harm. This may be challenging in terms of finding a balance between the need to preserve technical neutrality and temporarily having to become less neutral to protect the adolescent and the treatment.

Alertness to *countertransference* helps the interviewer maintain a neutral stance and provides information that can guide further questioning and interventions. The clinician's *interpretations* then integrate information that can be looked at jointly and safely from a new perspective, such as role reversals that can occur when split representations of self and other arise.

Clarification asks the adolescent to further elaborate on and develop his report of experiences of which he is conscious (Caligor et al. 2018). However, confrontation goes well beyond such descriptive demands; by simultaneously highlighting contradictions in thinking, it draws the adolescent's attention to the defenses he is using at the moment and the eventual recognition that how he was thinking/acting/representing his inner world was inconsistent and problematic and therefore not really adaptive. This realization can result in significant discomfort, which can be a desirable goal because it motivates the search for a new level of adaptation while also allowing the therapist to guide the discussion toward employing the cognitive skills that are now available to the adolescent and fostering flexibility in his thinking by bringing up alternative perspectives (i.e., different constructions of reality) for consideration—new ways for the adolescent to look at his experience, alongside the perspective that dominated his previous constructions. In effect, the therapist guides the adolescent to self-reflect, and by helping him step back from what had been an automatic style, helps him become aware of his inconsistencies, leading to a realization that this style is no longer adaptive or adequate and that a new level of adaptation needs to be found. The adolescent, with his newly developing capacity to deal with complexity, develops the wherewithal to recognize that different constructions of reality can be considered simultaneously (e.g., "let's suppose that…") and that keeping constructions (i.e., dyads) separate, each in their own compartment, is inadequate and is likely basic to his problems. This paves the way for interpretation, which offers a greater level of self-understanding (Caligor et al. 2018).

# Case 2: Jonathan

Jonathan was an anxious high school senior who, functioning primarily at a neurotic level of personality organization, provided an opportunity to utilize confrontation when he presented two contradictory self-representations. In one, with regard to classmates, he indicated that he felt disrespected, ignored, and left out of activities or at least not sought. He emphasized his dissatisfaction that he was more passive than he wanted to be, and he understood this in terms of his anxiety with others. For example, he was eager to go on a date and attend his class prom but could not imagine mustering the courage to ask a girl out. He did interact with girls within the classroom context. Alternatively, he provided descriptions of himself acting in an assertive manner as an editor of a school publication. Consistent with his level of personality organization, his descriptions often provided a clear picture of his experience, and the therapist did not typically have to push for extensive clarification. Although he primarily resorted to repression-level defenses, a quality of splitting was seen such that confrontation remained a useful intervention. The therapist placed before him the two contradictory dyads—the passive, ignored, anxious one who is looked down on or ignored by others and the boss who gives orders to others, who typically listened to him. The discussions that arose about these contradictory self-images led to an increased awareness of his conflict about the expression of aggressive and sexual feelings and his ensuing anxiety. He resented this position and, reflecting healthy developmental urges, wished to be more aggressive and to engage in a range of relationships. In addition, movement in this direction would also reflect a step toward greater autonomy and reduced identification with his anxious father.

The therapist's confrontation highlighted for Jonathan that his feeling upset over passivity was the dominant experience of one moment that contradicted the dominant experience of being in charge and giving orders at another moment. Although the latter was his expressed wish, he had little awareness of the extent to which he was already doing this—that he had been recognized and appointed to a prominent role that required him to exercise power. Instead, he was more alert to his suppressed anger and discomfort when he thought his staff was noncompliant. The confrontation and ensuing discussions provoked reflections that contributed toward a reexamination of his sense of how he saw himself.

The impression is that this adolescent was holding in mind two contradictory representations of himself that were embedded in the separate expressions of his experience. He was most cognizant of the dominant representation of himself as an anxious, passive young man who could be upset with himself about his habitual restraint and avoidance. Although he could state, with minimal fanfare and no obvious pride, that he had a prominent role in the school publication, he seemed to have no awareness that in performing those duties he was exercising power and was responded to appropriately by many students. It was as though he kept each representation of experience in its own compartment, to be thought about individually and in isolation from the other.

## Case 3: Ben

Ben was a 17-year-old boy who showed significant features of a narcissistic personality disorder organized at a moderate to high borderline level. He had difficulty developing warm relations with family, friends, and teachers. He was committed to remaining in psychotherapy but consistently avoided the acknowledgment of any feelings toward the therapist. He could show significant anger in the family and hostility in other relationships. He was aggressive at home and in therapy in the form of yelling and hitting walls (while restraining himself from damaging the therapist's wall) but was not physically aggressive in other settings. He said he liked to use therapy to complain because he could not do it anywhere else. He would typically complain about his parents and siblings, presenting himself as the continual victim of their selfishness, unappreciated for how much he does for them and enraged by how they deliberately provoked him by doing the annoying things he asked them not to do. Several of these projections were consistent with the paranoid quality he showed when discussing others, especially teachers and classmates. Although he complained that his parents did nothing for him, he was aware that they said they had tried to buy him things and had asked him to join family outings and were frustrated that he would not let them make him happy. By avoiding accepting from others, he avoided feelings of dependency and fears of regression, thereby not engaging in behaviors that would promote greater independence and autonomy. He would complain about his parents and siblings at most sessions, for prolonged periods, and objected when the therapist attempted to curtail the complaints and engage in other discussion and interaction. Repeatedly, for long periods, the therapist would confront Ben with the contradiction between his current complaint and other things Ben had said or knew that indicated positive qualities in his parents. Quite often in the early phase of treatment Ben would ignore any statements about their positive features, but only later, coinciding with a decline in the paranoid quality to his thinking and representation of others, did he utilize the confrontations to pay appropriate attention to the positive and negative elements of his representation of his parents such that he could acknowledge that they were "good people" and that someday he would probably end up being like them, which he thought was a positive thing.

The therapist's confrontation attempts to shake up the system, to help the adolescent recognize that his current mode of adaptation is distorted, inadequate, and inefficient. Ensuing discomfort about this can raise awareness that a more adequate adaptation must be found. These contradictory expressions of the conflict may come up many times, but each confrontation, and the self-reflection it demands, promotes development toward a more adequate adaptation associated with a more mature defensive posture. A structural reorganization does not occur immediately and may be related to level of pathology. For example, the reflection and reevaluation of representations occurred more readily for Jonathan than Ben. Finally, the therapist does not portray an investment in either of the contradictory elements, thereby maintaining neutrality. Had the therapist shown, for example, a need to have Ben like his parents, then Ben would understandably see the therapist as an adversary who preferred Ben's parents.

# Interpretation

The stages of interpretation include 1) *clarification* of the adolescent's communication and trying to help the adolescent elaborate to increase her comprehension and reach the limits of her self-awareness before contributing with additional observations from the therapist; 2) *confrontation* involving tactful exploring, with the adolescent, of his nonverbal or other behavior; 3) *interpretation* and the formulation and testing out of hypotheses regarding the unconscious implications of what has been clarified and confronted: first in the unconscious meanings in the "here and now" and later in the corresponding unconscious meanings in the "there and then."

In TFP-A, *clarification* is a central technique because most adolescents do not yet have the same ease and facility as adults to think about, express, and communicate their affective experiences and concerns. The therapist thus plays an active role in helping and keeping the clarification going until the adolescent develops the capacity to do this with less and less scaffolding from the therapist. Adolescent patients with PDs frequently have a very limited sense of themselves and others and generally are inclined to focus only on the behavioral rather than the psychological. When working with such patients, some scaffolding gets this ability going.

The technique of exploring in "loops" what the patient thinks about what she has said, about the reaction of the therapist, and where the patient stands now regarding what she has said involves clarification in the sense of exploring the patient's conscious and preconscious awareness of her mental state. It is an essential technique facilitating the development and elaboration of the comprehension regarding self and others, or "mentalization." Clarification includes significant aspects of the patient's life outside the sessions; the use of patient expressions stemming from sources such as diaries, literary productions, or drawings; and the patient's description of her relationships with friends and important people in her life environment. The patient's enthusiastic wishes to tell about experiences she has had outside the sessions are encouraged to lead to detailed narratives within which the patient's reactions and reflections may then be explored.

Regarding *interpretation*, we generally start out very carefully with extratransferential interpretations—tentative efforts to link the content of different sessions—to establish a continuity of contents that originally may have been presented split off from each other, and these interpretations follow a combination of economic and dynamic principles. The *economic principle* refers to what is affectively dominant in each session, and this exploration of what is affectively dominant derives from the therapist's combined assessment of the patient's verbal and nonverbal communication and the countertransference. In fact, consistent attention to these three sources of information proves particularly important in adolescents, for whom, in the early stages of treatment, much of the information is carried by nonverbal behavior and the therapist's countertransference reactions. Affective dominance, therefore, may result at times in verbal communications by the patient but, equally often, in nonverbal communication and countertransference.

The *dynamic principle of interpretation* refers to the need to interpret from surface to depth, from the defensive sides of the conflict to the impulsive sides of it, a general principle of psychoanalytic technique that becomes particularly important in adolescents given the risk of patients receiving any new information brought in by the therapist as an authoritarian "brainwashing." It is important to start out with common observations by the adolescent and the therapist regarding the reality of a certain fact that the therapist then may develop in further depth. If, to begin with, no common element of thinking or appreciation may be found regarding an issue the therapist thinks is important, the interpretation may have to begin simply with the therapist sharing a view on a certain issue about which the therapist believes the adolescent may have a different view and to demonstrate the fact that two potentially incompatible views of that issue are possible. In general, analysis of the defensive function of a certain conflict is facilitated by the fact that defensive operations are closer to consciousness than are dissociated, projected, or repressed operations. Interpretation of the defensive aspect and its motivation, and then what it is defending against, can be facilitated by the therapist with a tentative, open-ended style of communicating his or her thinking, always sharing it as something to be examined in the same way as statements of the patient are examined. The sum total of what has been said makes interpretation a slow process and assumes a lengthy preparatory process. A hypothesis about unconscious meaning is only tentatively introduced once abundant evidence on the road to that interpretation has already been elaborated.

The structural principle of interpretation classically refers to the assessment of which "agency" of the tripartite model of the mind is in conflict with which other "agency," involving the relations between ego, superego, id, and external reality. The question becomes, Which agency is the seat of the defense, and which is the seat of the corresponding impulse? In the case of patients with severe personality disorders and identity diffusion, the conflicts between libidinally invested and aggressively invested, positive and negative, and loving and hateful affective experiences are expressed mostly in the dynamic of split-off internalized object relations that, in the case of patients with normal identity, become the components, respectively, of the tripartite structure. In the patients we are considering, defense and impulse are expressed in dissociated internalized object relations. Thus, an idealized relationship to the therapist may be a defense against a persecutory one, and that same persecutory object relation may emerge as a defensive function against another, positive internalized object relation, which becomes an impulsive one at a different time. The structural aspect of interpretations in these cases is therefore equivalent to the consideration of which object relation is dominant in the transference at a given point and the gradual sorting out of the self and object representations of that relationship and their interchange in the transference. Eventually, the conflict between impulse and defense is played out between idealized and persecutory transference relationships.

The following is a session with Jacob, a 13-year-old whose case was introduced in Chapter 5, in the context of contract setting, to illustrate the process of interpretation and the active, playful style of the therapist.

# Case 4: Jacob

In therapy, Jacob habitually slouched in his chair and seemed to turn off and become morosely silent and exaggeratedly tired and sleepy the moment he entered the therapy room. This contrasted sharply with how he behaved when the therapist first accompanied him from the waiting room, at which time he seemed evidently happy to see her, talking on the way to the therapy room about computer games, card collections, and television series and seeming obviously pleased when he could see that she knew what he was talking about. The main difficulty, however, was his extreme and prolonged silences during the sessions. Although it is common for adolescents to be silent, especially during the beginning phase of treatment, Jacob's silence went far beyond this. An intense paranoid reaction was apparent, and he acted like someone who had been dropped behind enemy lines. Jacob used his silence so that he could feel in control of the relationship. While this defended him from revealing and facing a much more sensitive, dependent side, it also left him with a very restricted, inadequate range of interpersonal responses and evoked frustration and rejection in others, who felt devalued and treated as though they were trying to control him. His peers did not tolerate his superiority and haughtiness, and they humiliated and rejected him when he responded in that way. He was highly sensitive to this but unable to defend himself from it, except through aggressive retaliation.

The following extract is from a session after a humiliating experience at a summer camp where Jacob's characteristic stubbornness and refusal to participate in any activity provoked mockery and rejection from the other boys. For example, he refused to prepare for a 3-day survival excursion, which could potentially place other members of the group at risk. He found the rejection by his peers extremely humiliating and difficult to tolerate but had no other strategy to repair and reinsert himself socially and consequently remained rejected and isolated. When he was no longer able to tolerate this situation, he phoned his father and asked him to come and fetch him. In this session the therapist uses clarification, confrontation, and interpretation to address the dyad that Jacob sets up with the therapist, in which he induces her to become the controlling object.

> THERAPIST: Do you have any further thoughts about the meeting we had with your parents?
>
> JACOB: No, but I guess we are obliged to talk about it. [The therapist had the impression here that this was said without hostility and that Jacob actually wanted to speak about it, but he would only do this in the context of an interrogation, a dyad wherein he was the victim and the therapist the torturer.]
>
> THERAPIST: Does it mean that you don't want to share your thoughts because you have the impression that I am forcing you?
>
> JACOB: Let's say, just as a question, what is your point in asking me? If YOU want to, we will end up talking about the meeting, about what you have seen. [He has successfully reestablished the victim/torturer dyad, even though the family session had ended with a feeling of cooperation.]
>
> THERAPIST: If I understand you correctly, you seem to think that I have something in mind and you will have to hear it no matter if you like it or not, no matter if you want it or not. It may be important to try to understand why you see it like that; either you are right, but then we have a problem because I am certain that you know that therapy is not about a therapist imposing on a person in need, or there is something in you right now that needs to see me as imposing my own point of view on you— [This is an attempt by the therapist to clarify in a manner that invites the patient to respond by offering him a choice. The patient chooses a third option—no response.]
>
> JACOB (*interrupting the therapist*): I have nothing to say!
>
> THERAPIST: Wait a minute, Jacob. Are you answering my first question or commenting on what I just said? Right now, I was questioning the fact that you stay with the impression that I am forcing you to talk, that you have no choice, and this situation leaves us with two options: either you are right, or this way of seeing me helps you in some way.
>
> JACOB: I have the choice to leave if I want…I also have the right to remain silent and sleep for an hour (*said in a somewhat haughty tone*).
>
> THERAPIST (*smiling*): Yes, this is right, and by doing that you can be freed from having to decide between the two ways of seeing the situation.

JACOB (*nodding, with a triumphant smile*): Yes!

THERAPIST: You smile, as if now you are the one who is in control of the situation, and of me.

JACOB: Yes!

THERAPIST: What I am wondering now is that, during the session with your parents, you were able to share what you have been experiencing at the camp and seemed to be able to participate in the discussion actively and honestly. I am wondering if anything has happened since then to explain why you seem now to behave as if I am against you. [The therapist is providing a confrontation.]

JACOB: I don't know; nothing has changed.

THERAPIST: This is interesting....Do you remember how you were able to talk during that session?

JACOB: No, I am the same.

THERAPIST: Right now could you say that there is a part of you that is convinced that I am controlling you so much so that you feel justified to not respond. I understand that. [The therapist offers an interpretation, with empathy, of the current interaction.]

JACOB (*looking more vulnerable*): But I have the right to stay silent, you just said so. What is the problem?

THERAPIST: Right now we are stuck, because you are so convinced that I want to control you or force you that you don't see any other possibilities but to oppose. This thought seems so strong that you even forgot how it was during that session and especially at the end of that session. It looks as if something terrible is going to happen between you and me. Do you have any idea? [The therapist offers an interpretation with a comment about defenses (forgetting).]

JACOB: I am sure that you will want to dig and dig and dig and find another fault.

THERAPIST: Aha! Again, this is quite interesting and I think we have to try to understand what is going on right now. What I understood at that meeting was that you had a good reason for not wanting to stay at the camp anymore, and that your parents didn't understand that. They were not able to understand the reason it was so difficult for you to stay at the camp. What I understood from what you were saying is that it was difficult for you to stay there because you could not bear to be humiliated for being French and being treated as different from Quebecers and put aside. You found it difficult to protect yourself and defend yourself. I don't think your parents knew that side of you, at least it is not a side of you that you show to them. Most of the time, they see quite a different side of you. It seems that there is a side of you that feels easily hurt, easily humiliated, and you are not able to protect yourself. And then there is that other side that acts as if nothing happened. (*Jacob remains silent but appears to be listening.*) When we look at what is happening between you and me right now, you seem to be engaged in a similar struggle with me. Because you are deeply convinced that I will find faults, that I will humiliate you, you don't have any other choice but to start a battle and being really decided to win that battle. But do you see how this side clashes with the one side at the camp who could not tolerate being joked at and humiliated? So, there is that part of you that is very "defiant," very "arrogant," as your parents would say, and that other part of you that is very, very sensitive, easily hurt, and defenseless. What do you think? Is it possible? [The therapist offers an interpretation that utilizes the transference.]

JACOB (*mumbling*): It's possible! I don't know.... Anyway, what is the problem?

THERAPIST: I guess we have a problem. I say "we," because I think that what happened at the camp is serious because it shows a part of you that needs help to learn to protect yourself. But when I offer my help, you don't see it like help; you have the conviction that I will humiliate you even more, that I won't let you say what you want to say, that I will do whatever I want with you, that I will force you to talk, that I will torture you. So we have a problem, because it seems like the only way you think you can protect yourself from me is to stand up against me. It is okay in a way, because I think you get some sort of a reassurance from that. It is like saying to yourself, "So it is me who is in control here, nothing will happen to me!" It is okay in the sense that you communicate something important there, but deep down, there is a problem, and the problem is that it is your only card. When you get into a situation like that—let's say with your parents—they react quite strongly when you enact this role, because you don't have any other card in your pocket. With your classmates, or with the other boys at the camp, you couldn't use that card, or maybe you used it, I don't know. But, am I right if I say that if you were inflexible with them, they would go away or they would continue to provoke you and hurt you?

JACOB: That is true. They were laughing at me.

THERAPIST: Your card, the only card you have in your game, which is to be opposed... to stand up...was not working there, and it left you exposed.

JACOB: Hmm... hmm... yes.

THERAPIST: Yes! I find you quite courageous for saying yes, like during the meeting with your parents, I also found you courageous for tolerating being there with them while they were obviously angry and depreciative of you. Courageous for staying there. You didn't subside into your chair; you didn't fall asleep. You did not provoke your parents too much. You were able to tell me enough about what happened with the boys at the camp and the issue around your French accent so much so that I could understand how difficult it must have been for you at camp. I found you courageous because you, in a way, admitted that it had nothing to do with finding the camp boring, that it had nothing to do with the fact that it was not what you were expecting. (*Jacob now looks engaged and interested.*) And I don't know if you noticed something then, but your father changed his attitude toward you just before the end of the meeting. He mentioned that you have expressed remorse for him having to drive all the way to the camp to fetch you and that you were searching somehow for ways to repair it by offering to pay for the expenses.

JACOB: I know, I remember...

THERAPIST [later in the session]: I wonder if we can understand that famous incident where you assaulted one of your classmates last fall. I wonder if there is a link between being unable to protect yourself when you feel humiliated and exploding? You know, between the fact that this person had probably provoked you by humiliating you and that the only way you could find at that moment to stop the torture, to protect yourself, was by hitting him. [The therapist provides an interpretation that goes beyond the moment and links events across time.]

JACOB: Yes, he did not want to stop. The girl, too, was provoking me. [The patient thus reveals that he had been assaulting at least one other classmate.]

## Time to Interpret

The question about when to offer an interpretation is important. The general rule is that the interpretation should be offered at the earliest possible moment the material makes it clear what to interpret. However, some adolescents are sensitive to ideas that come from someone other than themselves because they are in the middle process of constructing an ideal by their own that will guide their transition into adulthood. Any confrontation to their shortcomings and vulnerabilities may jeopardize that project. Other adolescents firm up their reliance on an omnipotent sense of self or project onto others their disowned self-experiences. Therefore, offering an interpretation without any warning or preparation can evoke anxiety and possible immediate rejection.

The general principle in TFP-A is to start from the surface and work toward the unaware or unassumed. One example is an adolescent who accuses the therapist of being dishonest while being patently dishonest himself or reacts with indignity if someone else lies. It would be inappropriate or risky for the therapist to say to the adolescent patient, "You attribute to me what you can see in yourself," although we may say this to an adult patient. The therapist instead may say, "It enrages you tremendously to be confronted with somebody who is dishonest. I wonder why so much? What is so terrible? Let's say I am really a dishonest person, I am a liar. What is so terrible about this?" The adolescent may respond, "It's terrible because you ask us to be honest while you, as an adult, act otherwise." The therapist may then say, "You talk as though you have been exposed to that a lot, that you know a lot about it," and then slowly add, "Have you ever been tempted to act like that, to be like that?" The adolescent may then confide, "Yes, why not? If adults do it, why not us? Why not me?" The therapist may then offer the following interpretation: "So, if I understand you correctly, it is infuriating to see that adults do what they want without remorse or punishment; for them it is okay, but with you it is a problem. It is not fair, it is unjust. In a way it entitles you to do the same things."

Another principle is to be "cost conscious" in interpretation. This is raised by the concern of therapists who are not sure what to interpret or who are looking for the right clue to enable the appropriate interpretation at a given moment, the interpretation that will bring about a shift of emphasis in the unconscious transference. Some therapists are more intuitive or quick than others to identify this clue. Paulina Kernberg taught that what matters to the patient is not the accuracy of the interpretation so much as the willingness of the therapist to help as well as the therapist's capacity to identify with the patient; to believe in what is needed, no matter how painful, disturbing, or choking it may be to the patient; and to meet that need by making the adolescent aware of it and offering an interpretation as soon as it manifests verbally or in nonverbal language. Therefore, a therapist should not have any hesitation in playing for time, by which we mean allowing himself or herself to be involved in an introductory or preparatory phase, playing, constructing with the adolescent, or just waiting and "looking useless" for the patient. This style reflects the epitome of being active with the adolescent patient.

## Playfulness and Metaphor Intervention

The use of metaphor facilitates mentalization capacities because it can mirror or evoke feelings in the patient in a way that facilitates empathic attunement. The feelings that are activated are more tolerable because the metaphor acts as a "trial identification" and can then be objectified, and thus its power to distress or overwhelm is mitigated.

### Case 5: Joelle

Joelle is an 18-year-old woman with BPD who looks like Marilyn Monroe—blue eyes, blond curly hair, a little chubby, and a goddess smile. She declares that she can take "any man in her bed," that no one can resist her. After leaving a residential setting where she had been placed for more than a year, and unable to live with her parents because she was "an adult now," she instead went to live with a 38-year-old man, an ex-convict who was just out of prison.

She mentions that he is an unattractive man but that she does not mind and even likes it, because no woman would be attracted to him. At the same time, she admits that she is not in love with him; she stays with him because he loves her and thinks that it is mutual. In her mind, however, the real reason she lives with him is because she does not have any other place to go and because it allows her the possibility to be involved with his 2-year-old daughter, to whom she has become attached.

She has come to her session anxious because she is convinced that her boyfriend is having an affair with someone else. Her understanding of the situation is that she has been seeing other men and having sex with them and that he must have become aware of it and is seeking revenge and wants to make her suffer. Although her understanding may prove correct, her lack of concern for him in the first place, her risky sexual behaviors with other men, and her self-centered reaction expressed in her fear of being kicked out of his apartment lead the therapist to focus her intervention on an antisocial dyad in which she uses others for her own benefit.

THERAPIST: Yes, it is a possibility; he may want to make you pay because, as you said last time, he loves you and is attached to you. By having an affair with another woman, he may want you to suffer, just like he does when he learns that you are having affairs too. But I notice that you seem to agree with that behavior. If you do it, why can't he do it?

JOELLE (*looking confused*): Yes, that is true, but what do you mean?

THERAPIST: Where are you surprised?

JOELLE: I was surprised that another woman can be seduced by him. Also, he used to say that he loves me, that he will never do anything to hurt me.

THERAPIST: So, you are surprised that someone may change his mind, he may have moved on, may do things that in other circumstances he would not do.

JOELLE: Yes, and now I am really concerned that he will kick me out of the apartment, and I do not know where to go. (*Bites her nails.*)

THERAPIST: In your mind, it looks as if it is more bearable to think that "it is a revenge" because it would have meant that he is attached to you. It can even allow for the possibility to continue to have affairs, because he is so attached to you that he will not survive if you abandon him.

JOELLE: Yes, I see what you mean.

THERAPIST: Realizing that "love" may fade away under recurrent attacks and disrespect makes you feel anxious, because you realize first of all that it may have consequences, but also that you may no longer control him and that you may be responsible for your own misery. It is like a "declaration of war." If a country feels that it has been attacked by another country, that conventional rules have been violated, no matter if the two countries were allies before, it declares war—not as a revenge, but to reestablish boundaries, respect, and autonomy. New sets of rules have to be agreed upon before the end of the war, otherwise the first country will make friends with other countries. The problem here is that continuing to think that he still loves you puts you into a fragile position—you risk being kicked out of his apartment without notice or having time to find something else. You're not protecting yourself when you have sex with strangers because you are more invested in "doing what you want." You feel entitled to do it because you don't love your boyfriend, as opposed to taking good care of and protecting yourself. And thus you do not have the opportunity to learn social rules that could protect you from living in chaos.

JOELLE: I see what you mean; I like the image of the "war." I understand now. It is a bit much for me though to swallow; I feel guilty now.

THERAPIST: Why do you feel guilty?

JOELLE: Because I realized that I am a "bad person," and it is not what I want. I do not want to be a "bad person."

THERAPIST: Guilt is quite an intense emotion; it's scary to feel it.

JOELLE: Hmm, hmm.

THERAPIST: I see…I understand why it may be difficult for you to respect rules and agreements, even between us. After our first session, you decided not to come back, even though you had agreed to. It took you 2 months to call me back and ask for an appointment because things were not going well between you and your mom. I offered you an appointment, but you canceled three times before coming, mentioning that you had to work, to go to the dentist, and the last time you offered no reason. I had to leave you a message that mentioned something like, "It looks like my good intentions to help you are not convincing enough to make you decide to come, or it may make you decide not to come even though it may look paradoxical. I really do not know which one of the two it may be, or for another reason that we won't discover because you are not coming. Therefore, I think it is best to give the appointment to someone else at this point. You could call me at a later point, when you will be able, or even not completely able, to control that urge to cancel our appointment or at least be prepared to explore it." It made you call me right away, and you have not missed any appointments since then. If I would have known you better, I would have said (*in a playful tone*), "I do not want to see you! 'Bye!"

JOELLE: Yes, it's silly, eh?

# Transference-Countertransference Analysis

As with adult patients, because of the strong predominance of negative transferences that are typical in the case of severe personality disorders, it is important to interpret both positive and negative transferences to avoid conveying the impression to the patient that she is "all bad." This becomes particularly relevant in the case of patients with severe narcissistic transferences, with their tendency to dismiss and devalue all of the therapist's suggestions. Pointing out, for example, the patient's capacity to be openly critical of the therapist as a way to stress the positive aspects of courage in her communications may be helpful to a patient who otherwise feels that she is always involved with a critical therapist.

Transference interpretation usually starts out with significant exploration of transference displacements to external figures. The interpretation of the transference in relation to the therapist may be opened as a "playful" invitation to the patient to express in fantasy and playful action in the session his experiences of or thoughts about the therapist. It is important to understand the patient's feelings in this regard in terms of the patient's developmental level. The therapist may make an appropriate bridging from play to verbal, symbolic communication of the meaning of the adolescent's experience and interaction. The therapist may suggest to the patient that acting-out behavior, as well as somatization, may at times express feelings that the patient would not dare to express toward the therapist. This represents another bridging effort to bring these manifestations into a verbalized, affective, and symbolic context.

In the case of severe paranoid regression, transference developments may emerge at a paranoid level at which reality testing is temporarily lost. The adolescent may develop hallucinations or transitory delusional transferences. In this case, the same method developed in TFP for adult patients applies here—namely, the analysis of "incompatible realities" in the transference. The therapist may have to suggest, from a position of technical neutrality, that she and the patient are obviously, at this point, living in incompatible realities and that this needs to be tolerated and understood.

*Countertransference*, in its contemporary view, refers to the therapist's total emotional reaction to the patient. It may vary from moment to moment in the sessions—an "acute countertransference reaction"—or be a long-term fixation and particular emotional stance regarding the patient, a "chronic countertransference development." The severity of the adolescent's acting out within and outside the sessions may promote strong countertransference reactions, reflecting both concern for the patient and fear that the treatment will be interrupted by the patient's behavior, which would not be tolerated by the parents and might provoke hostile reactions against the therapist. The intense, consistent dismissal and devaluation of the therapist's interventions by patients with severe narcissistic personality disorder may, over a period of time, seriously disturb the therapist's sense of security, raising intense feelings of failure and temptations to give up and the risk of losing sight of any positive transference manifestations. Among the most ubiquitous countertransference reactions to the adolescent are feelings that the therapist is a "better parent" than the actual parents, not tolerating aggression in the sessions and colluding with the adolescent, and feeling that the parents are overly critical or indulgent. Also, the adolescent's wish to maintain a dependent relationship with the therapist—despite constantly attacking the therapist—may be missed. Erotic countertransferences to sexually seductive adolescents may disturb a therapist more than corresponding countertransferences evoked by adult patients, stirring up profound oedipal prohibitions against intergenerational activation of sexual desire. Obviously, the therapist needs to tolerate these experiences—and neither act on them nor communicate them directly to the patient—in order to observe and come to understand them fully, using these reactions as material to be woven into transference interpretations. The general preparedness of the therapist to be alert to the risk of either adopting a seductive "freedom fighter" attitude toward the patient or becoming the "policeman" for inefficient parents should provide a general frame for maintaining an objective stance regarding countertransference temptations.

Sometimes the treatment is "blocked." Weeks of "non-understanding" or a pervasive sense of hopelessness may arise that interfere with the active work with transference and countertransference. Tolerance of such periods, with an openness to sometimes share with the patient the impression that the treatment has come to a standstill, may open up new information about transference and countertransference lines. Some adolescents have severe self-destructive tendencies and an unconscious tendency to destroy whoever tries to extend them a helping hand, as in the self-destructiveness of malignant narcissism, that may seriously limit the effectiveness of the treatment. We have to accept that not everybody can be helped with this treatment, or even with treatment in general. The major prognostic indicators, corresponding to those for adult patients, are the patient's remaining capacity for non-exploitative object relations, the absence of antisocial features and of secondary gain, and the patient's intelligence and demonstrated potential for creative functioning in some areas. A supportive family environment may be a major positive contributing factor supporting treatment with a very disturbed adolescent.

# Technical Neutrality

TFP-A promotes change by reactivating the internalized experiences of self and others so that the patient can begin to reflect on what he experiences and then connect this experience with internal representations that may not correspond to the external reality in obvious ways, such as what is happening in the present moment between him and the therapist. By maintaining technical neutrality, by not "taking sides," the therapist allows the adolescent to experience these intense emotions. For example, if he feels that the therapist prefers the parents' point of view rather than his own experience, he may stop considering all the factors that have an impact on his thoughts, emotions, and behaviors. On the other hand, technical neutrality must be implemented within a framework that also prioritizes threats and patient safety as well as normal development. Consequently, deviations from planned and justified neutrality are frequent in order to confront types of acting out that could endanger the adolescent, his development, or the treatment itself. For example, for William, the 12-year-old with explosive behavior whose case was discussed in Chapter 5, the prospect of being expelled from school could have important consequences for his development if it is the beginning of a vicious circle of expulsion and readmission. Also, admission to a psychiatric hospital could increase the risk of William's being labeled by others, and his seeing himself as having a psychiatric problem, while at the same time endangering his psychotherapy and the opportunity to gain a sense of his conflicts.

*Technical neutrality* has been defined as an intervention from a position that is equidistant to the sides of a patient's internal conflicts, as from the viewpoint of an "excluded third party" (Kernberg 2016). Technical neutrality implies equidistance from the id, the superego, the acting ego, and external reality and an identification not only with the observing part of the patient's ego but also with general humanistic values that favor and support life, respect for the individual, physical health, and emotional well-being. Technical neutrality does not imply a cold, rejecting, or uninterested objectivity but a warm, concerned, objective way of looking at the patient's internal conflicts. It is an essential position for the therapist in order to analyze transference developments credibly. It does not imply a lack of countertransference reactions, positive or negative, even intense countertransference reactions, as long as the therapist's interventions occur at a point where she has regained her internal objectivity.

Technical neutrality, as is the case with adult patients, may have to be abandoned temporarily when severe acting out threatens the patient's life, the treatment, or other people. The therapist may have to intervene with limit setting and has to be prepared to follow up over a period of time, fully exploring the reasons why technical neutrality had to be abandoned and the significance of the conflicts that were activated in this context, leading to the gradual analytic interpretative reinstatement of technical neutrality.

Structuring, limit-setting interventions that involve the patient's home, school, or social life may create significant and unavoidable complications to the therapist's efforts to reinstate a position of technical neutrality. In some of these situations, the therapist must also be alert to the possibility that the parents could see him as taking sides. Under conditions when the patient's sexual behavior, drug or alcohol abuse, antisocial behavior, or problems with the law require interventions from the parents, and these interventions may be complicated by authoritarian, even sadistic behavior from them, the therapist's efforts to maintain the structure of the treatment are particularly difficult; enormous efforts may be required to differentiate his interventions from the authoritarian behavior of the parents. It is a major challenge to maintain a careful equilibrium between respecting the privacy of the patient's sexual behavior and protecting the patient from dangerous expression of that behavior while keeping confidentiality and remaining within the boundary of legal dispositions. This challenge must be confronted while taking the minimum moves away from technical neutrality that protect the patient's well-being and the viability of the treatment.

# Developmentally Informed Interventions

## Separation-Individuation Anxiety

### Case 6: Bea

Bea, a 17-year-old, experiences severe panic attacks that prevent her from going outside of the house and therefore affect her school involvement. The therapist points out to the patient the impact of her problems on her developmental task, which is to move out of the safety and security of the home, and focuses her interpretative process on identifying Bea's "triumphant desire" to sabotage her life and control her parents.

Bea: Did my mother call you? I do not know if you received the message.
Therapist: I did not talk to her.
Bea: But she left you a message.
Therapist: Not that I know of.... What is it?
Bea: Last week—Wednesday, Thursday, and Friday—I did not leave the house. And on Friday, before I went to work, I put myself in a corner and did not want to move from there for about 20 minutes. I was shaking. Then my mother came in and found me.
Therapist: Excuse me, where were you?

BEA: I was in my room. It's a small corner between my bed and my library. It's not very big; I curl up in the corner.... When I do not feel well, I put myself in this corner, and I think... I was sitting in the corner, and I was shaking... I did not think. I was invaded... I told my mother that I never wanted to leave the house again. I wanted to stay there. I did not want to leave my room. Whenever I tried to leave my room, I had a panic attack. I tried for half an hour. I got up from bed, I went to the bathroom... I was so exhausted that I fell asleep on the floor.

Friday I could not physically go to the bathroom anymore. I felt like the walls were closing in on me. I needed to get out of there. I kept coming back to my room. I just wanted to hide in my corner. My mother found me there and took me to my grandmother's house because I did not want to be alone. She wanted to call you, but I told her you were on vacation. So she wanted to call Dr. Keats, but I had not told her—just as I had not told you—that I had missed some appointments with Dr. Keats. At the last meeting I had missed with her, we spoke on the phone. When she spoke to my mother, she said that I was no longer her patient because I had missed the last appointments. My mother replied that she did not know that; she could not had known it because I did not tell her. My mother looked very angry because she knew I needed to talk to someone. So, Dr. _____ agreed to see me. My mother literally begged me to go. She told me that my grandmother would accompany me, that she would take me to the doctor and that I would take a taxi back home. She said to me, "Everything will be fine, you will be safe after that." I did not feel safe at all, I felt sure of nothing. Every day I was worrying more and more since I was in my corner.

Finally I managed to see Dr. _____. I told her that I lied more and more, that it was possibly that which had brought me there. My biggest lie was that I had not finished my screenplay... that I did not start my screenplay... which means that I'm stuck and that I'm just going to have to tell the dean that I cannot write it... and I will fail the class. How will I explain this to my parents, that I will not be able to graduate, that I am missing three or four credits? I do not really want to graduate, but how am I going to tell them that? That's all in my head. Dr. _____ told me that maybe I could write the screenplay during the weekend. I said I would try. I've tried many times, but I come home and I cannot write the screenplay. After that, we talked a bit about what we're talking about here, like the fact that I do not want to go to school, that I do not want to graduate because that means that I will have to start my adult life. You know, to start this new phase of my life, which totally terrorizes me.

When I left her office, I felt a little better. Going out seemed easier, because I knew that my grandmother was there and that I would be with her and that if I needed anything, I could rely on it. And then, my mother called my grandmother's house. I talked to my mother. I told her, "Please, you have to come get me, I do not feel safe here." My mother asked, "Why?" I said that I did not feel safe. I told her, "If you want, I can take a taxi, but I just want to be in my house." She came to get me. On the way back, she said to me, "Today you completely drained me of my energy. I do not know what to do." I felt bad about that, but she said calling her to take me back home was selfish. I said okay, but I just wanted to be at home, and here I would feel better. I told myself, I'm going to wake up the next day and I'm going to do my schoolwork on Saturday and Sunday.

I woke up on Saturday morning; my mother shouted to me that my dad was there and that both of them wanted to talk to me. I came down, but I did not want to talk to them. I told them. My father said (for once in his life), "Bea, we're here for you. Every time you want to talk you just have to ask for help. Tell us if you need help so you will not end up in this state." I told them to leave me alone, that I feel attacked, that I did not want to talk about that at that time. I realized for the first time in my life that I had two sides in me—no, was not the first time, but it was obvious that time—one side in which I want to tell you everything, that I do not want to lie. Another side of me tells me to stay away, to lie, to continue like this. Unfortunately, this last side always wins. I do not know…my parents talked a lot. My mother said that she was very angry and that she had to call my father because she could not stand this anymore. She felt so lonely. And I felt so attacked throughout the conversation. And then, finally, I had to leave the room after they asked me if I had something to say. I told them no, and they asked me if I still wanted to leave. I said yes. Although they were so nice to me, I still felt attacked. After that, Saturday was pretty awful. I cried most of the afternoon. I stayed in my room and fell asleep until about 6 A.M. or 7 A.M. I got up; I talked to my grandmother. I hated the fact that she had phoned my father.

THERAPIST: Why, in your opinion, did she do that?

BEA: Because my father…he's a tough person when you have to talk. He always starts by being very attentive and affectionate (and this time, he was very much so), but that, one way or another, always ends badly. When he begins to speak, it ends always in a nightmare; I feel attacked most of the time, as I feel when you speak, too. I just wanted to talk to my mother. But when she got home, she was exhausted and just wanted to sleep. Finally, last night we talked; I told her about the screenplay, I told her about the school credits. She looked at me and said, "Big deal, Bea, okay, do not think about credits anymore, I'll give you the money." She was very supportive. I looked at her, and I asked her how it was that I was convinced that she would not support me— because she is really supportive. And even my father, Saturday he told me that "they would provide for me"—of course, I have to find a job, but they would take care of the apartment, the food—"Me and your mother are going to take care of that" and that's true…it's just that I always come to the conclusion that they will let me down. This was triggered by this dream that I had last Wednesday. I had a bad dream, a very bad dream that my mother would die. After she died, everyone left. It seemed so real, and I did not know how to take care of myself, and then big bugs replaced all the members of my family and my friends, and they wanted to catch me. That scared me, because inside, I'm still a little girl. Whenever I have all these fears, I told my mother that adult life frightens me. Also, I thought I was the only one living this, but now I think everyone is going through it.

THERAPIST: It's a paradox to be so scared about adulthood when childhood seems so scary too.

BEA: Yes, I know.

THERAPIST: I think you will not like what I'm going to say.

BEA: I do not know what you are going to say.

THERAPIST: Because you have tremendous power to convince yourself and to convince your mother, your father, and your grandmother that you are totally helpless, that you cannot do anything.

BEA: I'm not; I will not be.

THERAPIST: I think that you're almost trying to stop time, because that way, your mother will not change, you will not change, you'll stay like that for the rest of your life. You'll never lose anyone, no one will grow old, no one will die. I think you're coming…actively…you're getting into a state of stupor, you're convincing yourself and your family…when you're not taking your medication, when you're not sleeping.

BEA: No…

THERAPIST: You come to feel that if I did the same thing as you, I would feel a lot worse than you…just think of the isolation…I would feel easily depressed.

BEA: No.…For a while, when I went out, the only thing that comforted me was the idea of going home after work. After class, and even though I was very tired, I was happier going back home because it was comfortable.

THERAPIST: Yes, everyone likes to go home, because they will have time to rest.

BEA: It's different. I do not want to honestly be in the world, I want to be at home.

THERAPIST: But look what happens when you're at home: you're alone. There is a movie title: *Home Alone.* (*Laughter.*) I don't know what you like so much about it, an overdose of being at home.

BEA: Why?

THERAPIST: You have panic attacks, you cannot sleep…

BEA (*plaintively*): I cannot leave my house. I love my house.

THERAPIST: But you came out of the house; you went to see your grandmother to have company.

BEA: No, my mother sent me there.

THERAPIST: You are maintaining that state of mind. Anyway, it was not a very good experience to be alone at home. You want to keep thinking that it's good at home.

BEA: It's a love-hate relationship. This is the only place where I feel very comfortable, but it is also a place where I can become very destructive. I do not do my work, I watch the TV, I play video games.

THERAPIST: You are really destructive…but very destructive.

BEA: Exactly.

THERAPIST: You know, the reason I said you would not like what I was going to tell you is that you have these tantrums that you express internally rather than externally.

BEA: I can understand that.

THERAPIST: From then on, you can think that your mother…that you can ruin everything, that you can destroy everything. You act, you behave in such a way that you can put everyone in this situation. You have lied about your medication.

BEA: No, no…I take my Prozac. But maybe Dr. _____ will not want to see me anymore.

THERAPIST: But she saw you, didn't she? But you know, I start to doubt what you told me, because you told me you could not breathe: "I cannot breathe anymore. I almost became blue and suffocated because I could not breathe." If you are able to put yourself in a situation where you are going to feel "suffocated" (everyone would feel like that in such a situation), you are aware that you are doing toxic things.

BEA: At a level…

THERAPIST: You do toxic things to yourself and so you have the power.

BEA: I do not know what else to do.

THERAPIST: You know what to do, but you do not do it. You convince yourself of being powerless, while you have all the power to destroy yourself and destroy your relationship with your family. In fact, should we bring your mother? What do you think we should discuss with your mother, if she wants to come?

BEA: I do not know; she has already tried so hard.

THERAPIST: You want to prove that your father, your mother and I, and your psychiatrist, that we are, and your grandmother, that we are totally unable to help you while you—

BEA: That I am unable to help myself.

THERAPIST: No, no, that you are totally unable to help yourself. Fully capable of not helping you. You do exactly everything that is forbidden.

BEA: I cannot.

THERAPIST: How can you be so effective at not helping yourself?

BEA: I am…It's the only thing I'm successful at.

THERAPIST: Yes, and you smile while saying that.

BEA: That's the case, because inside I know it—it's the only thing I do well.

THERAPIST: Now, the question is whether your mother should participate in this game. That's why we need to discuss whether your father and mother should play in this. Because as long as you are going to believe that you can get support from your parents, or work that you do with me, only to prove that you will triumph.

BEA: I know, I sabotage; I do it all the time. (*Laughs.*)

THERAPIST: It is very important to discuss all of this here, but from the moment you use it to sabotage everything outside, our discussions give the impression of a drop of water, as if they are useless, because you continue to do it outside.

BEA: No, it helps.

THERAPIST: You continue, happily, to sabotage everything.

BEA: But do you understand that that part of me is stronger? It surpasses me.

THERAPIST: I'm more impressed by your power to…you create situations from outside, in your life, outside of your sessions here, so that, all happy, you make your mother's life hard, you make life hard for your father, you lock yourself in your room, while convinced that you are helpless. While me, what I see, is someone who has done a whole show, a play of gigantic proportions. The question now is whether your mother can help you not have all the power to do all these things.

BEA: But what should she do?

THERAPIST: We need to discuss with her how she feels she helps you sabotage and how you manage to make her do that. She may not be aware of that.

BEA: Oh no, she is conscious.

# Integration of Sexuality in the Self

It may be particularly important to focus on the adolescent's romantic and sexual life, an area that is a conventional cultural taboo in terms of communications between adolescents and adults and may emerge only in subtle, indirect ways, through sexualized behavior in the session, in erotic countertransferences, and in a clear discrepancy between the patient's sexualized behavior on the one hand and complete absence of information regarding erotic experiences and behaviors in the adolescent's external life on the other. The management of erotic transferences may present a difficulty in terms of showing up in countertransference reactions while the adolescent studiously avoids any reference to his or her erotic fantasy or behavior. Tactfully pointing out the erotic implications of the adolescent's behavior in the hour, and its contrast, with no reference to erotic experiences outside the hours—as though an important aspect of life were missing in the patient's experience—may bring the subject into full exploration. Here, direct, open discussion of sexual issues in a noneroticized context and without taking the side of "superego"-determined criticism or rebellious stimulation of "sexual freedom" unlocks this important area of the adolescent's life experience, including the difficulty with talking about sexual inhibitions, polymorphous sexual behavior and fantasies, and confusion and anxieties over sexual wishes or inhibitions.

Male psychotherapists may have particular countertransference difficulties in exploring sexual conflicts with female adolescent patients with BPD. A patient who has provocative, sexually seductive behavior, while consciously denying all interests or concern about her sexuality, may present the therapist with the conventional stereotype of the implicit seductive stimulation involved in an adult man bringing up sexual issues with an adolescent girl. Indeed, through the mechanism of projective identification, the patient may attribute such sexually seductive intentions to the therapist's intervention. Frequently, behind significant eroticization in the transference lies predominantly preoedipal issues, the need for attention from and dependency on a parental figure, rather than a direct expression of oedipal fears and desires. In cases of predominantly narcissistic pathology, erotic seductiveness may reflect the needs for admiration and desire by the patient and replicate the use of erotic attraction for omnipotent control that is expressed in external relations. In their relationship with female therapists, girls' provocative, sexually exhibitionistic behavior more often signals competitive rivalry and rebellion against frustrating and prohibitive maternal images.

For example, a 15-year-old attractive, very intelligent girl entered therapy because of her anxiety, primarily about school performance. However, she quickly began to talk about the boys at her school, whom she described as immature while also indicating that she found them interesting and enjoyed hanging out with them. She also described her mother's involvement, suggesting that significant secondary gains had resulted from her anxiety. She described her father as distant. Suddenly, at the end of a session, as she was leaving, the patient smiled and approached the male therapist, who was still seated, and patted him on the head. He noted his surprise and that the patting was more like one would do to a pet or a little child, like a controlling and controlled expression of affection that denied the reality of the adult male with whom she was meeting and the nature of their relation. This transference provided initial entrance to a subsequent discussion of this act, which led to further thoughts about her discomfort with her increasingly demanding sexual feelings and awareness of sexual interests and her conflicts about what to do with this in regard to the boys and her father.

# CHAPTER 7

## Tactics of TFP-A

**IN CHAPTER 5,** we specified the first tactic in Transference-Focused Psychotherapy (TFP-A), which is the establishment of an initial treatment contract with the adolescent and his or her parents, to address urgent difficulties that may threaten the adolescent's physical integrity or survival, and that of other people, and conditions that will guarantee the continuation of the treatment. After the usual arrangements of a psychodynamic treatment are stated, conditions under which the treatment can be carried out that involve certain responsibilities for the patient and certain responsibilities for the parent and the therapist are agreed on. What is important, next, is to implement the treatment within these stated agreements.

We present here a series of other interventions that maintain, in each session, the conditions necessary for working with the adolescent and for protecting the TFP-A treatment. These interventions include maintaining free association by the adolescent; identifying and focusing on the priority theme in a session and developmental challenges; selecting what to interpret; and managing resistances and negative therapeutic reactions, including affect storms, psychopathic transferences, acute and chronic risks, and suicide risk. We also discuss specific tactics concerning parents, including those related to managing confidentiality and parental guilt, and countertransference with parents.

# Interventions to Maintain Conditions for Working With Patients and Protecting Therapy

## Maintaining Free Association

Within each session, the adolescent is encouraged to speak freely about what comes to his or her mind during the session. If the patient remains silent, the therapist presents tentative thoughts about possible reasons that prevent the patient from talking freely. Here, it is important that the therapist not attempt to "guess" what is in the patient's mind, but clearly express tentative thoughts regarding potential explanations for that behavior, to be confirmed or disconfirmed by what the patient says, followed by a period of expectation for a response from the patient, and renewed stimulation afterward if the patient continues to be silent. If that stimulation does not produce any change, then the patient's "silent" reaction to the therapist's effort may be interpreted as part of what is going on in the session, and this cycle of stimulation, namely the "reflective loop"—waiting, interpretation, waiting, stimulation, and so forth—is continued, thus gradually interpreting the meaning of the nonverbal communication. This usually is an effective way of dealing with silences and exploring their transference implications.

The frequent stimulation of the adolescent in terms of what his or her reactions are to what is going on in the session and to what has been discussed, and the adolescent's thoughts about what has been happening in the session, are ways to stimulate the patient to explore his or her self experience and the experience of the therapist's interventions in the session. Following these interpretative efforts, raising the question with the adolescent of his or her understanding of why the therapist has said what he said, along with a repetition of certain subject matters in this reflective loop, may reduce the amount of material that can be taken up in each session; in fact, however, it increases the possibility of helping the patient to become aware of his or her mental states and of the mental states of the therapist, fostering the process of "mentalization." In the process, the therapist may evaluate the patient's self and object representations, their projections, the intensity of affect activation, and the extent to which the patient's cognition is framing his or her affective experience and giving evidence of the patient's developing reflective capacity and empathy.

TFP-A encourages this type of communication even though with younger adolescents it may be difficult to understand at first. There are different explanations for why it may be difficult for adolescents to consent to that technique: 1) it requires speaking freely in a face-to-face interaction, which is not yet developmentally sustainable; 2) it can induce paranoid reactions; 3) it reveals adolescents' confusion, which they are trying desperately to hide and be free from; and 4) it draws on reflective capacity and empathy, which may be challenging because many patients with personality disorder (PD) are known to show reduced capacities to mentalize, especially in the context of interpersonal interactions (this is even more of an issue at adolescence, when the brain is still maturing)

Younger adolescents (12- to 13-year-olds) may need to be reminded of the period in their life when they were playing freely, when their play was not planned but then turned out to mean more than what it looked like. Sitting at a table, face to face (or face to back), may also be necessary while playing at a board game, in order to relieve the tension of being too intimate. The therapist may say:

> Here, you know, is a place where you can say what comes to your mind. It is like when you were playing. At that time, you could use any toys you wanted, you could make any scenarios you wanted. At the beginning we may have had a slight idea of what the play was, but most of the time we wouldn't have been able to guess what it would have ended up to be. Here and now, my role will be to try to figure out what you mean and what it makes you feel, which may annoy you at the beginning because I may miss the point. Also, sometimes we don't want to say exactly what we think or we may not like what we feel, so we try to cover it up with other emotions or other tricks. Sometimes we don't even notice that we do that. However, if I notice it, I will try to help you to tolerate it a little bit more, and maybe we'll find together that it is easier than you thought. Am I clear to you?

With older adolescents, the free association technique may activate paranoid reactions. Some may think that it is our "special trick" to make them say what they do not want to say or, even worse, that we are in the pay of parents who want to know their secrets or deep thoughts. It is a "universal reaction" with an adolescent with PD, and it is especially noticeable in the beginning phase of the treatment. It compels the therapist to rapidly address this issue, which also involves a discussion around confidentiality and responsibility of the adolescent.

## Case 1: Robert

THERAPIST: Your mom is accompanying you?

ROBERT: Yes…I told her the other day that I was coming here but went to Fred. She learned it when you called home (*showing his discontentment*).

THERAPIST: You look as if I have done something wrong by calling your mom. Didn't we agree that because it may happen that you will not want to come, that in these circumstances you will make the effort to come anyway, even sitting in the waiting room, in order for us to have the chance to figure out what's happening. Am I right? Or did you change your mind? It is important to know, because this therapy may only work if you are here, even though I may sound silly by saying that.

ROBERT: Fred called me to say that he has something important to tell me…and he doesn't know that I see a shrink.

THERAPIST: Fred is the one who just dropped out of school and your best friend if I recall correctly?

ROBERT: Yes. But I did not want to come anyway.

THERAPIST: So, we are back to the agreement we had. You know that there is no reason for me to call your parents if you come (unless there is specific danger that you may be facing). Your parents agreed to this way of working together. So, there must be something else that I do not know or that I do not understand. Do you have an idea?

ROBERT: I agreed to come because I was forced to.

THERAPIST: How did they force you?

ROBERT: They would have forbidden me to play with my electronics. They wouldn't have stopped torturing me with that. I don't think that you know who they really are.

THERAPIST: So, if I understand you correctly, I was fooled by them as well as you. In front of me they agree to give you some responsibilities but did not mention that they threatened to take away your phone and computer, so it became a question not of coming or not, but of standing up for yourself, to let them know that even if your electronics are important to you, they are not so important that you would submit to their request. But you add something else—that you did not want to come anyway. What did you mean by that?

ROBERT: Are you going to charge my parents if I stay in the waiting room or if I don't come?

THERAPIST: Yes I will, because your parents agreed to that, and this agreement lasts as long as I consider that it is therapeutic. What I mean by that is that you may need some time to feel good and safe here or that you may act out some important feelings by not coming, like you did today. If we do not have the opportunity to talk about it, we will never know what those feelings or thoughts are, and you will lose a chance to learn to express them.

ROBERT: Oh! I see where you are going with that…if I speak more, you are happy and they are happy. But this is exactly what I do not want. I do not want you or them to know anything about myself.

THERAPIST: So you see me as more on their side than on yours? Now it makes sense why you don't want to come. Also, if you perceive therapy as an invasion into your "privacy," who guarantees you that I will not share it with your parents, especially since they could manipulate the therapist because I need their money?

ROBERT (*after a pause*): Yes! That's it.

THERAPIST: I may have a different perspective on that. Even though I take seriously what you think and believe, and this will need further exploration, it leaves us on "shaky ground." Am I like them or like any untrustable adult who says one thing and does otherwise? Or, am I greedy to the point of asking for your parent's money dishonestly? Or, and this is my main point, can I keep confidential material between us and therefore be strong enough to resist your parents' pressure? Can I be loyal to you? What am I obliged to tell them, and what can be kept confidential?

This adolescent with a schizoid quality to his defenses and interpersonal style, and consistent with his avoidance of whole-hearted engagement in school, peers, and sexual behavior, seems oblivious to the magnitude of his denial of affect and avoidance of overt expression of feeling. The therapist first may have to point out these qualities and indicate how they arose in therapy in reaction to certain questions as well as in this adolescent's silence merely from "not knowing" what to talk about. The therapist began to be alert to the adolescent's brief expressions of disappointment that were not followed by any expansive expression of affect, as well as to the therapist's own unfulfilled expectations that someone in this adolescent's position and intellectual level would automatically have more to say about the event in question. As a result, the therapist identified the need to guide the adolescent toward a recognition of what would ordinarily be expected at those moments, resulting in greater expression of content and affect from the adolescent. For other patients, a somewhat neutral interpretation of behavior and defenses might be appropriate. For example, the adolescent who begins each session and continues by constantly complaining about his parents prevents talking about himself and tries to force the therapist to take his side, perpetuating a "me vs. them" situation. The therapist might ask the adolescent if he has noticed that so much of the time is taken with his complaints about the parents that he is not offering anything new, and that while the adolescent might be disappointed that he feels he is not getting any help with his parents, it might be better if they talk more about him than about his parents. The therapist could then explain that such a shift would bring the therapy back toward the goals originally identified in the frame. A deeper interpretation of this adolescent's behavior might be appropriate as the treatment progresses.

However, how the resistance is manifested might also be indicative of the defensive style particular to the adolescent's PD and require somewhat more interpretation to move things along. As seen with Robert, a paranoid defense could contribute to a fearfulness about being exploited and a resistance to feeling controlled, in contrast to the power struggle and greater hostile, aggressive element that characterizes those with a more sadomasochistic defensive style. These forms of resistance would be in contrast to the resistance manifested by the adolescent with narcissistic features who expects to be treated in some special way and will devalue or demean the therapist. For all, the respective approaches would serve to maintain the status quo and support the secondary gains they receive from their pathology. The therapist might offer, "You seem to me fearful of telling me what your thinking about this…, as if I would then take this information and take advantage—use it against you in some way. It's as if it is hard for you to imagine that I might want to comment on it to be helpful. Let me remind you of what I said originally about how I do therapy, and in terms of today, in this case, I wanted to see if your comment could help us tie things together a bit, to work toward that goal of self-understanding; to see if we could move things toward your being able to think about yourself and not be fearful of what you discover—to be able to learn for yourself that you are not dangerous, not someone to be avoided, and nether am I."

The therapist's goal here is to create a setting where the adolescent feels safe to convey dominant, conflicted object relations that can be enacted, explored, and understood. In doing so, these procedures try to contain an adolescent's tendency to be active and to act out. Yet these procedures are not intended to be a controlling set of conditions; they should instead convey that the therapist has expectations about how adolescents could engage in their treatment while also encouraging them to meet their potential to participate in helping themselves. They are also intended to convey to adolescents that they will receive help and support in pursuing these goals. In addition, by being active in this way, the therapist is constructing a setting that helps contain his or her own countertransference and preserves technical neutrality.

# Identifying and Focusing on the Priority Theme and Developmental Challenges

A crucial tactical aspect of TFP-A is identifying the priority theme and elaborating this with a sharp focus on what is going on in the session itself. The selection of material to be explored depends on what is predominant in the adolescent's affect or, if that is not clear, what is predominant in the transference, or, if that is not clear either, what is predominant in the countertransference. At the same time, an awareness of the problems in reality that are dominant in the adolescent's life permits the therapist to intervene regarding these issues even in sessions in which affect dominance, transference, and countertransference do not appear clearly. A deviation from the contract or something new that might be a threat to the treatment is always given prominence.

A major emphasis in TFP-A is the attention to external reality—where the adolescent stands regarding his or her actual developmental tasks. How is the adolescent doing at school, at home, in social life, and with his or her personal well-being? Adolescents with borderline PD who are involved with drugs, alcohol, cutting behavior, and neglect of their self-care in daily life require careful monitoring of these behaviors and ongoing evaluation of their implications in terms of transference acting out. Transference analysis and consideration of external reality have to remain closely linked. In this regard, as mentioned before, the therapist's constant awareness of dominant problems in the adolescent's relation with reality helps to bring in those issues at times when intense transference-countertransference turbulence seems to direct the focus of the treatment almost exclusively onto what is going on in the sessions.

The priorities for interventions with adolescents are similar to those with adults and derive from danger signals that override the general criteria for selection of material to be explored:

1. Threat to life, particularly suicidal intentions or behavior.
2. Threat to treatment, represented by both refusal to come to sessions and indirect indications that the patient and family are considering its disruption.
3. Deceptiveness in the therapeutic hours, indicating a predominance of "paranoid-psychopathic" transferences that need to be explored. In general, chronic deceptiveness takes a high priority for elaboration over an extended period of time in some cases and regularly reveals underlying paranoid transferences: to openly "confess" certain issues the patient fears would create the danger of retaliation or punishment on the part of the therapist, parents, or other authorities.
4. Severe acting out, both inside the sessions and outside the sessions. Acting out usually indicates affective dominance of that subject and needs to be explored in the transference.
5. Trivialization. Sometimes, the only thing the therapist can diagnose is that the content of the hours seems to be trivial; there is no particular affect activation or affect "freezing," and both transference manifestations and countertransference dispositions are relatively quiet. The question

may be raised with the adolescent: What are we talking about? What is the relevance of all this? Are we leaving out important issues? In other words, the "looping" technique (reflecting on the recent interaction) (see Chapter 6) may be used to interpret the defensive functions of trivialization.

Here is an example on how trivialization has been addressed in one case.

# Case 2: Sophia

Sophia, a 13-year-old whose case was discussed in Chapter 5, was quite talkative, but the content of her speech was very superficial (e.g., talks about tricks that her dog does, visits that she made to the shopping mall with her mom, television shows that she watched when at her dad's). She never mentioned any difficulties at home (alcoholic mother, having been sexually abused by her mom's ex-boyfriend, serious custody issues between parents). She did mention during the assessment phase having problems at school—not liking anyone because everyone is mean and stupid—but never mentioned it again.

> THERAPIST: I see that you have lot of "good time" with your mom and also with your dad. That you like to be with them and like to be home. Do you sometimes want to be with friends?
>
> SOPHIA: No, I do not see my parents often enough. I spend one week with my mom and then one week with my dad.
>
> THERAPIST: I see that you like to remember "good moments." Is there time where you do not feel good at your mom's or dad's place?
>
> SOPHIA (*with a slight sigh of exasperation*): No.
>
> THERAPIST: You look a bit tense and uncomfortable with my question. It seems that it is important for you that you keep a good image of your family. It is not usually easy to live in two different homes and be able to have good relationships with two separated parents. How long ago were your parents divorced?
>
> SOPHIA: Five years.
>
> THERAPIST: Was it always that easy for you to keep good harmony with them?
>
> SOPHIA: Yes.
>
> THERAPIST: And your parents were also able to keep good harmony between themselves?
>
> SOPHIA: No!
>
> THERAPIST: It seems to be difficult to talk about it...also, I have the impression that by asking questions it forces you to give answers that you don't usually think about. You seem to have found a good way not to think about conflict between your parents: when you are with them, you are totally involved with

them, you like everything you do together, everything is geared at keeping everything under control, everyone happy. You are a little bit like that with me too. You talk only about subjects that are funny…nothing to disturb me or to displease me.

SOPHIA: But I do not know what to say. Maybe I should not say anything.

THERAPIST: It looks as if I have been blaming you for something terrible.

SOPHIA: Yes, you do not want me to talk about my dog.

THERAPIST: That is very interesting, I was questioning the reason why it is difficult to talk about your parents' conflicts, and I was impressed by your way of keeping them happy when you are with them, how it looks easy to appreciate small things that you do together to keep harmony. But if I point this out, you think that I am blaming you.

SOPHIA: I haven't said that I am always happy with them.

THERAPIST: Again, I am the judge, who looks for the fault or defect, and you are the guilty party who can only try to defend herself. Do you see what I mean?

SOPHIA: No, I do not feel guilty.

THERAPIST: But you feel me as someone who is judging you, who finds faults.

SOPHIA: Yes.

# Selecting What to Interpret

The general rule is to prioritize contents with affect that are expressed in the here and now.

# Managing Resistances and Negative Therapeutic Reactions

In TFP-A, we create a treatment framework within which it is safe to reactivate unconscious experiences and prevent the explosion of intense affects that darken communication. The therapeutic contract "serves to guarantee the scope of treatment, that therapy takes place on a regular basis and that patients can actively participate in therapy" (Yeomans et al. 2017). Means are regulated to protect against threats that, through the pathology of the patient, may endanger the treatment. As we have seen, the assessment phase gives the therapist an appreciation of what the threats to treatment may be, and the contract is the least restrictive set of conditions necessary to ensure an environment in which the psychotherapeutic process can take place.

Potential threats to treatment include, but are not limited to, severe self-destructive behavior with suicidal intent and other, more indirect behavior, such as when an adolescent becomes so angry at one of his parents that he begins to doubt the continuation of treatment. Resistances can constitute patient behaviors that generate external situations that endanger the therapy.

In the session, stubborn silence may be the counterpart of violent acting out outside the sessions, and the therapist may use the silences to point out that this reminds him or her of what is going on in other aspects of the patient's life. It is helpful to bring all communications the therapist has received about the patient into the session at the beginning of the session, to provide ample time to hear the patient's reaction to this information, inquire about the patient's view, and explore all its implications. Under conditions of significant paranoid transferences, deceptiveness, and extended silences, the consistent focus on nonverbal behavior may be very helpful to facilitate further work on the dominant transference-countertransference developments, with the therapist interpreting, first of all, the reasons why the open discussion of the corresponding conflicts appears to be so dangerous. The general sequence of *manifest behavior/defense → motivation for this defense → impulse need defended against* represents the dynamic principle of interpretation, complementing the economic principle of attention to the dominant affective content in the therapeutic hours.

## Affect Storms

The development of affect storms is a particularly frequent complication and tactical challenge in the treatment of adolescents. The adolescent should be free to express his or her affects in the hour as long as there is no physical attack on the therapist or the office or inappropriate sexual behavior during the sessions, and the patient's voice volume is contained by the office door and arrangements. It is important for the therapist to respond in affective terms that correspond to the affect activation of the adolescent, without the therapist entering into yelling matches or impulsive affective expression. In the case of opposite developments, with severe affect freezing and inhibition, the therapist has to be prepared to gradually interpret the transferential implications of that development as well. At times, severe affect freezing is a defense against the potential of a strong affect storm.

A major tactical task, at times, is to systematically analyze acting out outside as well as within the sessions, in order to transform it into a cognitively framed emotional experience that can be shared and jointly explored in the sessions. By the same token, the transformation of severe somatization into an equally shared cognitively framed affective experience that can be explored in the transference is an application of the same principle. Splitting processes in adolescents often take the form of a dissociation between severe acting out, on the one hand, and completely "nonrelated" affective reactions (anxiety and depression), on the other. For example, an adolescent may present with, on the one hand, serious failures in school and gross neglect of work that threatens him or her with academic failure, with no apparent concern and worry about it, and, on the other hand, nightmares, frightening dreams, and unexplained anxiety without any apparent content. Here, the major task is to overcome the mutual splitting of acting out and its corresponding affects, often linked with other defensive operations such as severe denial of the potential destructive effects of the acting-out behavior, and the unconscious enactment of guilt over competitive, self-assertive, or sexual gratification.

Unconscious guilt feelings related to oedipal conflicts frequently are condensed with preoedipal sources of aggression around frustrated dependency and abandonment. Although the adolescent may be able to advance into the establishment of a romantic love relation in which he or she has highly gratifying sexual experiences, unconsciously a price has to be paid, as represented by failure in other areas of his or her life, and this is evident in affects that cannot be traced directly to any conscious experience. It is extremely helpful to always ask adolescents who communicate that they feel anxious and depressed but do not know why about apparently unconnected behavioral developments that may provide the clues to the corresponding unconscious conflict. Sometimes the use of a metaphorical narrative, in which the therapist tells a focused story that reveals the conflict that has been dissociated in the separation between affect and acting out, permits the adolescent to realize what the issue is in that story and then to reflectively apply it to himself or herself.

## Psychopathic Transference

A particularly difficult situation may evolve with adolescents who combine deceptiveness in the sessions, what we call "psychopathic transference," with intensely paranoid developments and acting out, with multiple secrets distributed among family members, friends, and the school network, and the therapist, in turn, receiving "secret" information and intense concern from the family. Under such conditions, it is important to maintain ongoing contact with the family and open communication with the patient about the information that the therapist has learned, as well as to raise questions about information the therapist feels may have been withheld from him or her. The patient may run out of the session, enraged, or the parents may be enraged with their child or with the therapist, as "last ditch" protection against assumed threats connected to such "secrets." It is important to give an adolescent the choice as to whether he or she wants to participate in a session with enraged parents or prefers that the therapist meet with them alone at first, and only then jointly. Parents may become reluctant to remain firm in demanding that their child attend the sessions.

Open communication in those cases may be helped by the inclusion, at times of crises, of home visits by a "third party"—namely, a psychiatric social worker, teacher, or another member of the family. At times, efforts to structure the home situation with the assistance of, for example, a psychiatric social worker may be needed to stabilize the situation before further work can be done. It is important to differentiate clearly psychiatric social work as support for the psychotherapy from "family therapy," which may, in fact, be contraindicated in work with many adolescents with borderline PD, in which the patient's individuation and ability to function outside the home take precedence. Family therapy may sometimes have regressive effects for the patient and split the transference. In contrast, sophisticated psychiatric social work, with good coordination between psychiatric social worker and therapist, may restore or maintain an endangered treatment structure.

One important tactical problem is the development of negative therapeutic reactions—that is, when the patient experiences himself or herself as getting worse when in fact important positive developments have taken place. Such reactions have to be differentiated from negative transferences. One cause of negative therapeutic reaction is unconscious feelings of guilt over improvement; another important one, typical for narcissistic personalities, is unconscious envy of the therapist's very capacity to help the patient. The most severe type of negative therapeutic reaction is the patient's unconscious identification with a sadistic, battering object, particularly in cases of severely traumatized adolescents who have developed the fantasy that only somebody who makes them suffer really is interested in them. Another cause of apparently negative therapeutic reaction may reflect a reaction to some parents' inability to tolerate the patient's improvement.

# Acute and Chronic Risks

As with adults, adolescents with borderline PD may experience high levels of suicidal ideation and repeated self-harm. Therefore working with adolescents necessarily requires active engagement in the management of both acute and chronic exacerbations of risk. Acute and chronic risks may require different approaches. For example, a hospital emergency room may provide time-limited intensified support during a period of heightened acute risk. Yet in response to a less severe increase in risk, the same service may promote more active engagement of the adolescent in problem solving rather than providing more service input. Specific agreement to manage acute and chronic risks has to be negotiated in the contract.

Therapists need to be able to not under- or overreact to crises. They must remain alert to the potential dangers of reinforcing behavioral escalations with increased input and involvement and to the risk of withdrawing prematurely during periods of apparent stability and calm. The therapist must also take care not to ignore or minimize risks. Failure to respond appropriately to high-risk behaviors may result in behavioral escalations that cannot be ignored.

## Suicide Risk

In patients with chronic suicidal behavior, the fact that Transference-Focused Psychotherapy (TFP) focuses so importantly on the responsibility of the patient either to go into a hospital or to control the suicidal behavior until it can be discussed in the next therapeutic session may be difficult for the parents to tolerate. Here, extended meetings with the parents and the patient to explain the rationale for the maintenance of technical neutrality and for sharing responsibilities for the patient's survival and physical integrity with the patient himself or herself may provide the space for full explanations of the therapist's approach.

The development of dissociation between sexual behavior and the capacity for intimate love relations and tenderness may create a significant problem in the case of some adolescents, complicated further by the danger of sexually transmitted diseases and pregnancy. The main therapeutic tasks here are to untangle the condensation of oedipal issues with preoedipal aggression and to address the expression of sexuality as reflecting attachment needs rather than the integration of tenderness and eroticism. For example, a frequent constellation is an adolescent girl's search for a dependent relation with an adolescent boy by entering into a sexual relation that is perceived and carried out mechanically, or as a way to express unconscious guilt over rage regarding rejection. Some girls with serious limitations in their capacity for social relations become desirable to boys during puberty because of their sexual endowments, leading to disappointing, confusing, and traumatic early sexual involvements that require therapeutic work to facilitate the reintegration of sexual behavior and the capacity for intimacy with its developmental oedipal implications.

The complications of treatment in TFP-A derived from the comorbidity of eating disorders, drug abuse and dependence, and alcoholism are similar to those in adult TFP. Eating disorders may require parallel medical and dietary control and reeducation; drug and alcohol abuse has to be differentiated from substance dependency, and dependency may have to be treated simultaneously with or predating the treatment with TFP. If the psychotherapist expert in TFP is at the same time an expert in the treatment of drug and alcohol dependency, these treatments may be combined; otherwise, in our experience, it is preferable that the adolescent patient first be treated with detoxification and rehabilitation regarding drug or alcohol use, and only then receive TFP treatment. In the case of drug or alcohol abuse but not dependency, TFP should be able to explore and interpretively work through the acting-out functions of substance abuse.

In the case of dissociative reactions, it is important to differentiate severe PDs from posttraumatic stress disorder (PTSD). Here, much unnecessary confusion may derive from an overextension of the concept of PTSD, which, ideally, should be reserved to the typical syndrome that evolves somewhere within the first 6 months up to 3 years following an intense trauma. Physical abuse, sexual abuse, and chronic witnessing of physical or sexual abuse may be an important etiological factor in the development of a severe PD, but this etiology has to be differentiated clearly from PTSD proper because the treatment is completely different. In the case of PTSD, the treatment includes the possibility of reexperiencing repeatedly the traumatic situation within a safe, controlled therapeutic environment that permits its gradual elaboration and working through, often with the combination of psychopharmacological (anxiolytic or antidepressant), treatment. In contrast, when severe sexual or physical abuse is an important etiological feature in the treatment of severe PDs, it usually is reflected in the unconscious double identification with victim and perpetrator, and both types of internalized split-off object relations need to be permitted to evolve in the transference in order to gradually resolve them within the general strategic integration of identity.

The manifestation of severe acting out of aggression in the transference, sadomasochistic transferences, and the syndrome of "arrogance" (a combination of arrogance, "pseudostupidity," and curiosity) require the same technique of full elaboration and working through of the negative transference in the context of a clear protection of the boundaries of the treatment situation and protection of patient and therapist from any harmful expression of noncontained aggression.

The treatment of dissociative reactions follows the general principle of strategic resolution of severe splitting of self and object representations. Each dissociative state is explored as the activation of a particular relationship between self and object representations, and the mutual dissociation of contradictory dissociative states is analyzed in terms of the defensive effort to split primitive idealized from persecutory internalized object relations. Patients' attempts to treat each dissociative state as totally separate, unrelated to any other emotional state, experience, or conflict in their life, may raise anxiety and intense negative affect when any integrative interpretation is offered. This reaction, in turn, may need to be interpreted as the fear of bringing together love and hatred, ideal expectations and deep frustration and resentment. Respectful treatment of the patient as, at bottom, the same person throughout all the dissociative states contributes importantly to the tolerance and eventually resolution of these conditions.

One final, important tactical aspect of therapist interventions is the use, as much as possible, of the adolescent's own language to refer to his or her affective experiences and social relations. The adolescent may use a language with implications that are unknown to the therapist and that seem to have a defensive function without it being clear what exactly is implied in that verbalization. In such cases, it is helpful for the therapist to ask the patient what it means when he or she uses such an expression, and to express a willingness to then couch the corresponding affective experiences within that language of the adolescent. This may powerfully help the adolescent to open up to further exploration of his or her affective experiences.

The effective integration of the patient's self-concept and his or her concept of significant others—that is, the development of a normal ego identity corresponding to a normal adolescent developmental stage—will facilitate the adolescent's resumption of normal psychological growth. It will also show that the optimal features of TFP-A are not educational or reeducative efforts but a restoration of the adolescent's internal capacity and freedom to grow and develop creative relationships in work, love, friendship, and social life.

# Specific Tactics Concerning Parents

Consenting to a treatment, and even to an asessessment, is sometimes a complex process. The adolescent's high dependency, lack of autonomy, and vulnerability to parental pressure may leave him or her in a state of uncertainty depending on the degree of differentiation or conflict between the parents and the adolescent or between the parents themselves. It is therefore important to have an idea of the pressures that parents may have placed on the adolescent that may put him or her at risk of not consenting. It is common for parents to interfere with treatment, through either intrusions or even attacks, which may generate paranoid reactions in the therapist.

In some other cases, the parents actively debilitate the therapist as effectively as the adolescent can do through their lack of consciousness, insensitivity, selfishness, or tendency to exploitation. Parents can also actively contribute to adolescents' difficulties by misunderstanding their needs, inappropriately restricting their freedom, requiring them to take care of younger siblings while neglecting them, or exploiting them through de mands (e.g., requiring the adolescent to pay for costs related to his or her drug addiction).

In these cases where the parents present with severe pathology, the therapist should evaluate if it is realistic to try and work with parents, or whether it is better to focus instead on trying to help the adolescent. It is necessary to clarify what is the minimum that should be expected of them. Sometimes it is essential to involve the health care network, including social/child protection services. Most of the time, the adolescent must be helped to "separate" from his or her parents and be confronted with their sadness about not being able to "save the family."

# Case 3: Sylvia

Sylvia, a 13-year-old diagnosed with borderline PD with significant self-destructive behaviors, begins to pressure the therapist to recommend that she be admitted to a day hospital. Although her symptoms have improved significantly and there is adequate therapeutic involvement, the patient threatens the therapist with self-harm. The therapist tries to contain Sylvia's projections and help Sylvia to observe her own behavior. In one of the sessions, Sylvia exclaims, "I don't want to live anymore, I'm sick of everything, I've tried to ask for help and no one listens to me, my teachers, parents." It is clear that although the patient fails to mention the therapist, the complaint is clearly addressed to him. He is the therapist who does not behave as she wants, and she cannot tolerate it. The fact that the patient fails to control the therapist intensifies the pressure for the parents to take action. The parents turn to a private hospital to which they have privileged access because of the adolescent's suicidal behavior. In this way, they do not have to wait.

It is necessary in this situation to work with parents to help them understand their concerns about being unable to control their child's behavior and being afraid of his or her threats. Without the complicity of the parents to contain this situation, it becomes impossible to maintain the treatment, given the risk that the parents will act by interrupting the treatment.

In such a long treatment, parents often try to change the setting. It is essential for the therapist to convey to parents that they can call and speak with him or her before making a decision in the face of difficulties. Doing so can contain the parents and help them not to act. By working with the parents, the therapist can help them understand the importance of preserving the therapeutic space. In the case above, when Sylvia realizes that her parents have changed their minds and have stopped attending the private center, she resumes her binge eating, vomits, and inflicts superficial cuts. The therapist succeeds in restoring contact with reality and notes that the patient is angry with him and tries to attack him. Without the intervention of the therapist with the parents, Sylvia would have had the sole option of continuing this disastrous plan and might even have thought that the therapist was afraid of the parents and was unable to face them. A more resilient adolescent could also interpret the situation as one in which the parents have a strong power over the therapist, so the therapy would be doomed to failure.

## Managing Confidentiality

Normally, the therapist establishes a confidential and private setting to provide a therapeutic space in which to facilitate the deployment of dyads or triads of primitive object relationships in the adolescent's reaction to the therapist. These primitive object relations are the vehicle for the expression of intrapsychic conflicts that, in turn, are the subject of the interpretative process in TFP. However, if this framework is perceived to be threatened by parental intrusion or by the therapist's disclosure, a level of suspicion is introduced into the adolescent mind that permeates the transfer. Consequently, the therapist's efforts are aimed at resolving the intense negative transfer triggered by external reality as well as intrapsychic conflicts. Moreover, the adolescent could perceive this threat as a sign of infidelity and treason and then react by "sweeping the therapist," a destructive attack.

## Confronting Parental Guilt

Parents who seek consultation about their children, especially when severe relational difficulties and acting-out are involved, have often used the mental health system for a considerable amount of time and have often experienced judgment, disapproval, and guilt. As a result, they are often quite defensive and sometimes can be attacking and devaluing of the therapist as a way to protect themselves. Unless these attacks are confronted and interpreted as linked to their fear of being blamed again, it is difficult to consider with them the adolescent's problems and their own contribution to those problems.

# Management of Countertransference Toward Parents

Contemporary psychoanalytic literature considers countertransference as the set of emotional responses of the therapist to the patient at all times (Auchincloss and Samberg 2012). As we have seen, parents often interfere with treatment, through either intrusions or attacks, which can lead to paranoid reactions in the therapist. The therapeutic contract agreed on with the parents and the patient helps the therapist to be aware of these countertransference reactions (Yeomans et al. 2015, p. 176), as we have seen in the clinical vignettes presented in this chapter.

# PART III

Processes and Applications

# CHAPTER 8

# Phases of Treatment

**TRANSFERENCE-FOCUSED** psychotherapy for adolescents (TFP-A) can be conceived as having a beginning (preparatory) phase, a middle (core) phase, and an advanced (termination) phase. Although these three phases are not clearly delineated, and for some adolescents they may take more or less time to be achieved, we can recognize certain characteristics of each phase that can be used to follow the evolution of the treatment. Being aware of the main tasks that define each phase, as well as the clinical and technical issues that distinguish them, can help the therapist conceive the tasks that are expected at a specific phase and preview the expected clinical developments over the course of the treatment. It can also help to identify moments when the treatment regresses or stagnates.

In this chapter, we provide an overview of the three phases of TFP-A and discuss the clinical issues that typically arise in each phase of treatment.

## Beginning Phase

Compared with the treatment of adult personality disorder (PD), which formally begins only after assessment and contracting have been completed, the beginning phase of TFP-A is more crucial and, in some ways, more complex. It involves different members of the family, each of whom has different and sometime contradictory motivations and levels of implication, as highlighted in the assessment and contracting parts, but with whom the therapist will expect to have to deal in a collaborative way.

The following are the major tasks of the beginning phase of treatment:

- Implementing the treatment frame
- Forging a collaboration with the parents and reducing interference

- Forging a therapeutic alliance with the adolescent
- Stimulating mentalizing and fostering open communication
- Working with acting out
- Working with treatment resistance and paranoid transference
- Dealing with trauma integrated in the personality
- Identifying markers of change and transitioning to middle phase

# Implementing the Treatment Frame

TFP-A treatment proper begins after the assessment is completed, feedback is given to the adolescent and the parents/caretakers, and a contract is formulated that spells out the roles and responsibilities of the adolescent, parents, and therapist. It is important to be alert to any early breaches in basic contract agreements—for example, failure to maintain regular and timely attendance or payments. The therapist's goal is to create conditions that will promote the acceptance of TFP-A by the parents and adolescent as an individual psychodynamic psychotherapy that concentrates on working primarily with the adolescent to help with the concerns that brought him or her to treatment. To reach this point, it is often necessary to work with both the adolescent and the parents to identify their respective needs that could interfere with meeting the initial goal of forging an alliance with the former and a collaboration with the latter.

The biggest challenge at the beginning phase of treatment is addressing the fear of both parents and the adolescent that the therapist will try to control them. For the adolescent, the control theme often centers around issues of autonomy and may present as a need to control others in order to promote control of the self and a sense of independence. For parents, the control may present as a need to make things positive so that others (e.g., school, authority) will not try to control them and make them feel inadequate; in so doing, they may unconsciously resist what they experience as the therapist's attempt to control them. Some parents may also believe they must have a certain level of control to maintain a meaningful role in their child's life. Each may feel, as a projection, that the therapist wants to control them and, until they establish a sense of trust in the therapist and the process, may worry that the therapist is doing the other party's bidding—the adolescent may worry that the therapist is paid and controlled by the parents and is therefore merely an extension of them to also be resisted, whereas the parents may worry that the therapist is being fooled or manipulated by the adolescent, just as he or she has manipulated everyone else.

The danger for the therapist is getting caught in the middle of enactments around control, which, when not recognized, may result in frustration, anger, and attempts at supportive work to alleviate each party's complaint about the treatment, the therapist, or the other family member. As a result, the therapist is at risk of breaking the frame and losing technical neutrality. Instead, it is more fruitful if the struggles around control can be recognized and explained to the parties as another manifestation of some of the problems that brought them to treatment and of the way in which they manage certain fears. The explanation should be followed by an attempt to reinstate the frame as a way to approach management of the issue. It is valuable for the therapist to be alert to possible countertransference in these situations, such as identifying with the adolescent as a victim of the parents. The therapist may also experience a form of splitting in which he attempts to become the good child who appeases or satisfies the parents or the good parent who is flexible and thereby gets the adolescent to comply through kindness and care so that he will be liked. Becoming the parent may have an inadvertent seductive element that can have a counterproductive effect. None of these roles is therapeutic.

Once these issues around control are resolved, possibilities to establish a more collaborative mode of interaction with the parents as well as the adolescent open up. Hawley and Weisz (2005) determined that parent-therapist and adolescent-therapist alliances have different implications for treatment outcome. The parent alliance predicted therapy participation, whereas the adolescent alliance was the better predictor of symptom change. Thus, a strong alliance with the parents is important for treatment continuation, but alliance with the adolescent is more critical for treatment outcome. These two important alliances will be discussed in the next two sections.

# Forging a Collaboration With the Parents and Reducing Interference

Parents may differ from each other in how much effort is needed for them to reach an adequate understanding of their adolescent's problems. Forging a collaboration with the parents should help them 1) appreciate the seriousness of the problems so that they can move from denial or disavowal of the problem and from vague assertions of "behavior problems" to a realistic recognition and understanding; 2) move away from collusion in which both the parents and the adolescent have sought to minimize the problem; and 3) transition from a magical belief that things will somehow just get better to an understanding of why TFP-A is recommended for their child's particular serious problem and the implications of not pursuing treatment on current and possibly future functioning.

Sometimes, in their zeal to help their child, parents will take ownership of the problem—for example, intervening on the child's behalf with the school about uncompleted work or paying off the adolescent's credit card debt when the adolescent promises that "it won't happen again." By removing responsibility from their child, parents deprive their child of the "problem-solving experience," creating a sense of entitlement about what is owed to the adolescent and, perhaps most importantly, moving to quickly eliminate their own anxiety and discomfort. When this happens, the adolescent no longer has to feel her own anxiety. It should be felt, however, and the adolescent needs to develop the sense of control and confidence that comes about when one takes action that reduces one's own anxiety. In effect, this parental intervention maintains the parents as the strong, competent, controlling other, while the adolescent may experience herself—or believe that the parents perceive her—as weak, inadequate, and unable to take care of the business of adolescent life. At the same time, by continuing this pattern of behavior, the adolescent switches roles and becomes the powerful one who can make the parents anxious and make them do things to please her so that the adolescent will not be angry with them. These are the moments that parents experience themselves as "walking on eggshells" because they fear what might happen if they do not appease their child. This cannot be an effective intervention, because in order to remain powerful and controlling and to maintain this object relation for reducing or managing anxiety, the adolescent must continue to act in an inadequate manner and to show poor judgment.

Some parents, in collusion with their adolescent, seem intent on maintaining the status quo while continuing to blame each other, as though that is their only way of maintaining their relationship. This collusion draws the therapist into the parents' orbit and thereby prevents the therapist and the adolescent from forming the alliance necessary for the individual psychotherapy. Often the therapist must clarify the frame with regard to what he or she will be doing with the adolescent and why the current situation threatens the treatment. In addition, an empathic attitude by the therapist helps to prevent the parents from feeling castigated and provides an opportunity for an educational intervention that explains the situation within a developmental context while offering the parents an understanding of alternative actions on their part.

However, if the treatment is beset by repetitive variations of undermining themes, even though the parents seem to be trying to cooperate, it may be necessary to consider that the parents should see their own therapist to work with them on parenting skills or that the adolescent, siblings, and parents should obtain separate family therapy. Special situations, such as divorce, may make such an option more likely. The nature of the divorce, depending on whether it is hostile or cooperative, can have an impact on the treatment. The divorce agreement about custody and medical-legal responsibilities can affect the parents' participation and support in the treatment. The goal is to try to extricate the adolescent, the therapist, and their treatment together from parental, individual, and couple dynamics.

# Forging a Therapeutic Alliance With the Adolescent

The alliance begins to be built at the initiation of contact. As the adolescent describes his understanding of himself and his problems, he should be met with empathy and understanding in a nonjudgmental manner. In this way the adolescent may get to see that his pathology as represented in the contract has not been imposed on him—it is not derived from some "universal checklist" of adolescent problems—but is based on what he has been telling the therapist about himself. This can result in a discussion of why these actions present a problem and why they compromise his further development. This approach can help adolescents identify their own goals, which enhances the meaning of the therapy for them. Creating such a transition is important because adolescents with borderline PD are often referred by others (e.g., parents, school officials, social agencies) and may have different goals or no goals at all.

The recognition of therapy processes and parameters has a developmental progression (Russell and Shirk 1998), and the therapist must be aware that the adolescent's causal reasoning is still maturing and her egocentrism is only beginning to decline (Elkind 1967). This may limit her ability to understand the link between specific therapy tasks and subsequent therapy goals (Shirk 1988). We recognize that identifying long-term therapeutic goals and conceptualizing the link between such broad, often abstract goals and the more concrete session-to-session tasks of therapy are cognitively complex operations, and these types of reasoning skills are still developing. It may be necessary to accept that the parents and the adolescent have different goals and to help them be understanding and accepting of the other's perspective. These features also involve a sense of future, and the time diffusion described by Erikson (1968) that is associated with identify diffusion can be relevant. Some adolescents have the sense that things will take "forever" and that they cannot wait so long, because they are driven by the need for immediate gratification. Alternatively, others may feel that they have all the time in the world, so "what's the rush?" The parents may have a different time perspective that, although it may be understandable, may also be unrealistic for some change processes.

The greater the personal meaning of the therapy to the adolescent, the less likely he is to experience the treatment as part of a power struggle with his parents or the therapist. Goals may include stopping self-cutting, forming better friendships, or making school feel like a more comfortable space (not just getting better grades). A contract goal might be to eliminate risky sexual behavior; a personal goal might be to form a more intimate, romantic relationship that would include safe sex. In effect, the attempt is being made to sustain or enhance the adolescent's autonomy, but within the context of responsibility—that is, recognizing the motivating effect of excitement and coupling it with judgment so that the excitement eventually becomes a source of pleasure and satisfaction rather than a stimulus for worry or shame and concern about getting into trouble. Progress at integrating autonomy and responsibility implies improved self-reflective ability.

Most adolescents in psychotherapy can acknowledge having problems and can identify therapeutic goals (Garland et al. 2004), so the issue may be to define the problem in a manner that the adolescent can understand so that she sees the consequences by herself and for herself. Such an understanding can lead to treatment goals that feel understandable and not threatening to autonomy. Similarly, a therapist who is overbearing about the contract can create a threat that activates autonomy concerns. It is recommended instead to explore with the adolescent the possible meaning of her oppositional stance to contracting or its specific components and not to emphasize her "defiance" or reasserting control. This exploration may help her obtain insight into the anxieties that have been activated by entering the treatment and experiencing the transference. If effective, this would also give the adolescent an early taste of how therapy works and its potential to be helpful. The therapist is not omnipotent, and discussing this reality may have value. A therapist's concern about displaying strength may reflect countertransference that needs to be recognized and understood so that the adolescent does not experience a challenge to which she will feel a need to react.

Young people at a level of neurotic personality organization appear fairly comfortable in the therapeutic relationship. It is not unusual for these adolescents to play a role in initiating the request for therapy, and they are more comfortable than adolescents with borderline PD in asking for help or advice and in speaking about their ego-dystonic concerns and therefore feel safe experiencing a degree of dependency in the therapeutic relationship. Their discomfort is more about feeling the pressure of or expressing their inhibitions related to sexuality, aggression/competition, or separation and less about the therapeutic relationship itself.

Adolescents with borderline PD can experience considerable difficulty forming an alliance with the therapist. For these youngsters, feeling safe while experiencing dependency and regressive pulls, acknowledging a wish for help, and accepting what is being offered are very difficult. Because of the paranoid defensive style that so often characterizes adolescents at the initiation of therapy, and can endure for a while, they may not trust the therapist and find it hard to believe that someone could want to help them or give to them with no strings attached and actually be able to help them when they themselves often feel so overwhelmed. They may also have a concern about others' envy if they are perceived as being the object of someone's nurturance, as well as feel guilt about receiving it. These themes of dependency/nurturance and the associated fear of regression appear to enlist, often with greater frequency or intensity, the defense of omnipotent control that these adolescents often deploy in this phase of therapy. Also, the grandiosity they typically deploy is incompatible with attempts to establish the mutuality required in an alliance. Two clinical examples in this manual (see Chapters 1 and 4)—namely, the adolescent who needed to see the therapist as a "brick wall" (Case 2: Chris) and the one who devalued the therapist's comment by asking for the source of the interpretation (adolescent with mid-BPO)—illustrate these defenses against experiencing closeness with the therapist that characterize a narcissistic transference. These actions need to be approached by interpretation—by expressing to the adolescent the object relations that these defenses represent. However, these themes often are repeated and can go on for some time.

Other forms of early acting out that test the frame and the contract and prevent movement toward forming an alliance include missing sessions, not talking, or exacerbating symptoms that especially upset the parents. We emphasize interpretation with a focus on the feelings that might drive these behaviors and invite their expression within the therapy session rather than outside. This "invitation" is an especially important feature. It conveys to the adolescent, through the use of clarification, confrontation, and interpretation, that the therapist is also welcoming that part of him that he often feels is rejected by others, and that the therapist understands he has aggression—indeed, rage—but that the aggression, too, is an accepted part of him. This communication of the acceptance of an often split-off, projected part contributes greatly to the establishment of a sense of safety and trust with the therapist in this setting.

# Stimulating Mentalizing and Fostering Communication

Many adolescents with BPD may initially struggle to engage in a therapy that requires them to mentalize and put their experiences into words. This may be for two reasons. Compared with neurotic individuals who are able to communicate about their psychological experiences in a coherent narrative, individuals with PDs often have huge challenges in organizing and mentalizing about their experience due to identity diffusion. When combined with the adolescent phase, the challenges to mentalizing are even greater because many adolescents have not yet developed more mature reflective capacities and may have had little opportunity to reflect on their psychological experiences.

For many adolescents who come to treatment, it may be the first time they are invited to talk about and express their feelings and thoughts and think about their psychological experience and share this with someone else. At the beginning of treatment especially, there may be a learning phase during which the therapist helps the adolescent learn this language by imagining the adolescent's experience, clarifying and scaffolding possible understandings by putting himself or herself in the adolescent's shoes, sharing how the adolescent may have felt and wondering how the adolescent experienced the situation. The adolescent usually responds to this implicit invitation of the therapist and in a way uses this "squiggle" of the therapist to nuance and individualize the narrative. They may say, "No, it was kind of but not exactly like that. I felt more angry."

The young person's ability to focus and reflect on the therapist's comments will vary. These types of interventions, aside from the content in the therapist's comment (i.e., the meaning of the behavior the adolescent is asked to reflect upon), draw the adolescent toward reflection on internal processes rather than behaviors (i.e., what he was thinking/feeling, not just what he was doing). Although they may sometimes be able to be reflective in more emotionally neutral moments, the tendency of adolescents with borderline PD to be impulsive, take risks, act out, pursue more immediate gratification, and be influenced by expectations of peer reactions, all in the presence of incompletely mature neurocognitive control mechanisms, indicates the importance and difficulty of moving them away from action and toward reflection. The process does not emphasize the mere inhibition of the acting out but sees this behavior change ultimately as being the result of the effort to promote structural change. However, for this to happen, limits must be set so that the discussion can take place under safe conditions that are not dominated by the adolescent's threat to himself or to the treatment.

# Working With Acting Out

The need for limit setting by the therapist or the parents is not necessarily restricted to the beginning phase of therapy but may be more likely during this phase. As noted, acting out is initially dealt with by reviewing the contract with the adolescent and trying to identify what object relations are being reflected by her action. Thus, the contract does not eliminate the problem of acting out but provides one means for trying to contain it as the therapist helps the adolescent understand her self-defeating impulses and reflect on the meaning of her behavior. This approach may also convey to the adolescent, both directly and indirectly, the belief that she can take on greater responsibility for self-control, including the contradiction between her complaint that she does not want parents or others to control her while also behaving as though she were not fully able to control herself. Each of these interactions contributes toward establishing conditions that foster exploratory treatment.

As an "expert," the TFP-A therapist may present the adolescent with information about the maladaptive impact of his behaviors—for example, the impact of social isolation or the effect of lack of sleep and irregular eating habits on mood, attention, and memory. Of course, many adolescents will have already found counterarguments on the internet, such as may occur in a discussion of marijuana use in which they argue that heavy usage is safe and does not promote early onset of serious disorders, despite what research has shown. The problem can be constructed as follows: will the adolescent take charge of the care of his body and become self-nurturing, or will he engage in further destructive activity that negatively affects his ongoing development? In doing so, the therapist has in mind that the content of many of these games and animated cartoons is aggressive, and without this form of escapism the adolescent would have to face the issue of how to deal with his own rage, which the game and cartoons have been helping him avoid. The therapy then offers the adolescent the space to work on this rage as part of his work on how he feels about himself and others. This is an important element, because it may not be possible to feel worthy, to take in good, and to self-nurture if one experiences such rage and an urge to destroy when provoked.

# Working With Treatment Resistance and Paranoid Transference

Adolescents are typically ambivalent about confiding in the therapist. They fear that by doing so they place themselves in a compromising position in which the therapist can use their confidences to control them in some way or inhibit their striving to become independent, to have their own ideas, and to make their own decisions. More so than with adults, silences of this kind early in treatment often reflect patients' habitual defensive operations in a hostile world; in a way, it may be their only way to assert their authority.

It is important at the beginning of treatment with an adolescent to attempt to clarify the meaning or functions of the adolescent's silence. Often, the silence represents a transference resistance in which the patient immediately projects on the therapist his or her problem at home or at school. Prolonged silences may represent severe paranoid regression in the transference; in its most extreme form, silence becomes a form of acting out that defends against awareness of an overwhelmingly negative, paranoid transference. Both must be differentiated from the more conventional silences representing reflection, transference, and resistance seen in the setting of a strong alliance. The therapist has to use all the information that is available to attempt to clarify what may be motivating the patient's silence.

We begin by pointing out to the patient that he or she is silent. We wait a few minutes, then make another attempt to communicate our understanding of the silence, and we continue to evaluate the situation, including what is going on right now. This is to say, we alternate between tolerating silence and interpreting silence as it increasingly appears as the dominant issue in the session.

The therapist has to work very hard to try to understand what is going on while tolerating uncertainty. The therapist's ability to tolerate uncertainty is reflected in the therapist's somewhat tentative tone and attitude, which permit the adolescent to identify with the therapist's effort of not "knowing it all" while at the same time sharing. By portraying the uncertainty, the therapist helps the adolescent to tolerate that he or she does not always have to have the right answer in order to avoid looking foolish.

Within an object relations theory frame of reference, we can say that the therapist is, on the one hand, working to identify the paranoid object relation that is organizing the patient's silence while, on the other hand, introducing a different object relation. This provides the adolescent with the opportunity to identify with a specific representation of the therapist as trying to understand while tolerating not knowing it all and having that be known by the other. We do not always want to push quickly through the silence. Sometimes the silence may serve a holding function, in the transition between the acting out of the early paranoid transference and verbalization. As a result, it may take longer to say anything, not because we think the silence has any value in itself, but because it may take more time to figure out what is going on. Therefore, the therapist must not feel under pressure to stop the silence; he or she may wait patiently until a potential cue or interpretation arises.

In sum, the therapist has to see the work of silence as an interactional process that has to be analyzed gradually in all its components, in contrast to seducing the adolescent by making comments such as, "Why aren't you talking to me?" or "I am interested."

# Dealing With Trauma Integrated in the Personality

The fact that many adolescents who come for TFP-A treatment have a history of sexual traumatization and also some enduring PTSD symptoms raises the question of how to deal in TFP-A with trauma when it has become integrated in the patient's personality, as opposed to treating PTSD as an isolated syndrome. We differentiate the impact on personality functioning of trauma that is integrated into the personality from PTSD.

To summarize, the treatment of PTSD provides the patient an opportunity to revisit and relive the traumatic situation and its implications in the setting of an understanding, empathic, and safe relationship with an empathic therapist. The therapist helps the patient gradually work through the trauma while sharing with the patient all the feelings, anxieties, shock, disgust, and fear involved. With this approach, we treat the patient as a victim, and we help that victim overcome the trauma, keeping in mind that a trauma wakes up all sort of conflicts. Guilt feelings may come up: "I should have done something to prevent it"; "I must confess that I got excited." In other words, we normalize reactions of this kind, pointing out that the normal reaction to such an experience is a mixed one of terror, fear, and pain and sometimes also of pleasure; sometimes a sexual attack produces an exciting reaction or a feeling of being special, and the patient has no reason to feel guilty about that. We also focus on the reality of the attack in a relationship of trust and confidence.

However, when sexual traumatization is part of the etiology of a PD, things are more complicated, because we see a structural change in the personality as a result of the trauma, with the introduction of a pathogenic identification with both victim and aggressor. Thus, the trauma leads to the internalization of a highly pathogenic object relation of abuser and victim that, in the patient with borderline PD, must be kept isolated, or split off, from any positive relation and relegated to a highly paranoid domain of experience.

In TFP-A, the patient is unconsciously identified in a relationship, which means that he or she identifies with both the victim and the perpetrator. The patient reactivates this relationship in the transference. This means that the patient reexperiences and enacts not only the experience as a victim, but also the unconscious identification with her abuser. Thus the patient not only experiences the therapist as a new, dangerous seducer, but also, at the same time, often will herself become sexually seductive. In TFP-A, we work with the patient to accept these identifications with both the victim and the perpetrator.

The specificity of Transference-Focused Psychotherapy is to pay attention to the alternating identifications with self and object, victim and victimizer in the transference. With adolescents, when we see that the trauma has been integrated into the personality, we are likely to see its impact on the patient's sexuality. The trauma contributes to increase the power of split-off persecutory relationships and reinforces the recruitment of sexuality to the service of aggression. Sexuality comes to be used to attack either the object or the self (self-punitive, sexual humiliation) or to protest against the family. It is integrated into the personality structure.

# Identifying Markers of Change and Transitioning to Middle Phase

By the end of the beginning phase, the adolescent should have been able to identify and clarify his or her own personal goals of the treatment. The object relations that organize the adolescent's moment-to-moment experience and presenting problems will have been identified and agreed on. A collaborative alliance will have been established between the parents and the therapist in order to protect the therapeutic space. The adolescent will be more able to tolerate the experience of "free association" and sharing internal thoughts and feelings. Indeed, the negative transferences associated with having to trust a therapist while at the same time being aware of exchanges between therapist and parents, or with having to expose scarcely and imperfectly their intimate thoughts, desires, or feelings and risking feelings of humiliation, have been worked out.

# Middle Phase

The middle phase of TFP-A typically lasts 12–18 months, sometimes longer, depending on the family or social supportive system, the severity of the pathology, the need to temporarily suspend the treatment in order for the adolescent to gain confidence in her new abilities, and the level of autonomy attained by the adolescent that may motivate her to pursue longer. The beginning phase is marked by a reduction in suicidal behavior and self-injury, a decline in impulsivity and inappropriate behaviors outside the treatment setting, an increase in the capacity to experience intense affect in session, and the development of a curiosity about internal processes. These occur as the adolescent accepts the treatment frame, limit setting is effective, and expression of affect shifts into the therapeutic relationship, which allows for the active use of TFP-A techniques that promote further exploratory work. The decline in outside storms may co-occur with the increased expression of strong affect within the sessions. For all this to take place, it is essential for the parents to comply with the frame so that the initial levels of acting out outside the therapy are not maintained and reinforced.

The central task in the middle phase is to explore and work through the object relations that are defining the core conflicts in order to integrate split and dissociated self and other representations. The following are the major tasks of the middle phase of the treatment:

- Working from extratransferential material to transference
- Integrating split object representation and negative affects
- Consolidating other dimensions of personality organization
- Doing active work on countertransference

## Working From Extratransferential Material to Transference

With the adolescent, the treatment proceeds at first by using the TFP-A perspective to explore extratransferential material. This initially provides a sense of distance and safety for the adolescent, and he is less likely to feel "invaded" while exploring his strong affect in a setting with the therapist, who is offering comments and asking the adolescent to become more aware of and to work on the inconsistencies and incongruities in his thinking and perspective of others. The exploration of pathological object relations in this material paves the way to focus more on the transferential relationship and engage with the most immediate here-and-now experience.

The narcissistic transferences that were more prominent earlier in the treatment may become an area that the adolescent can now reflect on. Earlier, she might have rejected the therapist's attempt to be helpful and might often have shown this by immediately commenting that the therapist's comment was wrong (e.g., "No, that's not right"; "Yes, but…"), including a follow-up statement that might have been similar to the therapist's. Thus, she struggled to acknowledge that she was being given to—that the therapist was knowledgeable and bore some responsibility for her improvement. She needed to be the one to solve the problems and move things along, otherwise there could be no movement. In this next phase, the adolescent can reflect on the therapist's statement, "Have you noticed that whenever I would comment, you would tell me I was wrong?" She would not be expected to accept blame for this or apologize; instead, she would move toward greater openness, with increased receptivity and less omnipotent control.

# Integrating Split Object Representation and Negative Affects

Attempting to integrate the split object representations receives increased attention in the middle phase. These pathogenic object representations reappear and continue to be identified. The adolescent with borderline PD may continue, but with less frequency and intensity, to devalue the therapist by pointing out that "you already said that" or "you told me that already." He can be asked what he makes of this observation, and this moment also provides an opportunity to explain (and reexplain) that this is what happens in the therapy process and "will probably happen again." Devaluation of the therapist (implying that the therapist is stupid or old and cannot remember what was said or is young and does not know anything) may occur to offset the adolescent's embarrassment that he continues to do the same thing (i.e., make the same mistake) and the worry that the therapist may think that he is not smart or is a bad patient. The educational component lets the adolescent see that these problems (or the structure behind them) come up in various ways across situations, and the repetition may leave him better prepared to handle it when it occurs. Clarification and confrontation are continued, and the conflicts that initiated the reappearance of these object representations are examined. This process and an object relations perspective can be applied to the examinations of aggression, sexuality, their interaction, and other themes.

Improvement, reflected by increased integration (decline in splitting), may be illustrated by an altered representation of parents. For example, one adolescent constantly complained about his parents. He just wanted to continually "vent" about them in his sessions and portrayed himself as the victim of inept, uncaring parents who constantly treated his siblings better than they treated him. Over time, he could acknowledge that they were "good people" and that he was, in fact, like them in values and goals. However, developmental pressures to move forward toward greater separation and autonomy would evoke anxiety and a shift back to venting about how awful they were. A greater degree of integration of positive and negative representations was still needed in order to tolerate the warmth and closeness he felt, and his rage may have served to prevent experiencing guilt about his wish for this closeness, thus preventing a move to a more depressive position.

A different picture may present itself when parents are truly neglectful. Some parents of adolescents with borderline PD cannot or will not change and struggle with parenting and fulfilling the contract because of their personal pathology. They may tell the therapist to change their child, basically just dropping her at the office, but it is to their credit if they promote regular attendance. In such a situation, it may be of value to help the adolescent recognize the flaws in her parents and not have to maintain the self-image of the "bad one" in order to preserve an image or hope of the good parent. The adolescent thus may come to identify the love she feels for her parents while also recognizing the parents' negligence or antipathy.

# Consolidating Other Dimensions of Personality Organization

Sexuality, moral issues, and narcissistic struggles are explored after the main dyads have been analyzed. The reason for this is the importance of consolidating different elements of personality organization at this sensitive period of adolescence. The process involves interpretation to facilitate awareness and integration.

For example, Thiffany, 17 years old, started treatment after three suicide attempts. She also engaged in self-mutilation behaviors and had a moderate eating problem involving, for example, restricting her food intake or refusing to eat for a number of days. She has a long-standing history of emotional negligence by her two alcohol-dependent and immature parents, who separated when Thiffany was 7 years old. Her mother worked as an escort and her father was violent toward Thiffany's mother and always had financial problems. Thiffany was sexually abused by her paternal grandmother's husband (not her biological grandfather) from the ages of 9 to 13. At the beginning of the treatment, the main technical difficulty was that Thiffany was silent most of the time, did not elaborate any thoughts, and looked frightened and fragile as if anything could break her. After a year of treatment, the split parts of herself were becoming increasingly integrated, and her aggressive impulses were much more tolerated and accepted. She fears trusting or depending on someone and also fears what will be discovered in the treatment, She hides her rage under her fragile appearance because she fears that she could become as aggressive as an abuser and, if that were to happen, would hate herself as she hates the abuser. At the same time, she is struggling, in the treatment, with a more resistant object-relation dyad around dependency and the integration of sexuality into a mature self. She begins to experience the therapist as an "idealized object" who should always be there when Thiffany is depressed, scared, or stressed, otherwise she becomes infuriated and wants to punish the therapist. At a deeper level, much more unaware and unassumed, she also experiences the therapist as a "perverted object" who has to be seduced to get attention. This last aspect is manifesting in a disorganized, childlike seductive and sexual presentation such as wearing a provocative dress, when usually she wears normal clothes.

# Doing Active Work on Countertransference

During this phase the therapist focuses on identifying the dominant affect, as well as the prominent and hidden dyads. As this work becomes increasingly complex, the therapist must use all the different channels of communication, including verbal as well as nonverbal and countertransferential. The countertransfer enables the identification and elaboration of the different poles of the dyads, for example aggressor-victim.

In summary, the middle phase of treatment is characterized by more stability, and the focus of the interpretive work is on internal psychic processes, key conflicted object relations, and negative affects in concert with an increased capacity to self-reflect on transference and extratransferential dyads. Psychic integration increases with reductions in splitting of objects into idealized and devalued extremes. The result is the emergence of new, more integrated ways of seeing the self and others, Also, other facets of personality organization, such as sexuality, moral system, and narcissism, are more consolidated.

# Advanced Phase

In the advanced phase of the treatment, the dominant object relation dyads activated in the transference between patient and therapist as well as with external persons are more easily recognized and acknowledged. Particular attention has to be paid to the extent to which regressive attitudes of the adolescent have changed in favor of a greater degree of reality and taking responsibility. Calls for the patient to express himself about the therapist and his thoughts can provide indicators on the extent to which the young person is capable of changing perspectives and thus has made an important step toward integration.

The following are the major tasks of the advanced/termination phase of the treatment:

- Gaining self-awareness that projection and splitting distort reality
- emergence and development of new self-reflective capacities
- consolidation of personality structure

## Gaining Self-Awareness That Projection and Splitting Distort Reality

The adolescent becomes aware that their perception of people and experiences is influenced by their emotional states and their particular way of projecting their conflictual drives on others. For example, during this phase the adolescent starts to see their parents in a more nuanced way. The result is a more realistic and balanced view of people that leads to improved relational functioning and a capacity to invest in developmental tasks.

## Drawing on the Emergence and Development of New Self-Reflective Capacities

The advanced phase is characterized by the emergence and development of a more nuanced and balanced sense of self and others in which the adolescent is able to appreciate both the positive and negative qualities of themselves and other. Gradually they become more able to reduce projection and splitting and develop a capacity to hold on to the sense of the other as also having good qualities, even when they are frustrated by others. Having an increasingly balanced representation of self serves to break the destructive cycles of splitting and the escalation of negative affect that cause inappropriate interpersonal behaviors and undermine relationships. As a result, the adolescent has the opportunity to stabilize their relationships, and in turn, develop a sense of their own stability.

In this phase, when growing reflective capacities are available, interpretation has a different effect, and the adolescent can better use it for self-exploration and the capacity to identify and block projections.

## Moving Toward Consolidation of Personality Structure

The developments outlined previously and the integration of personality are associated with an increasing awareness of aggression toward others and the hurt and damage this may have caused to loved ones. This may trigger a depressive reaction that is important to address. It is important to address this development through clarification and interpret it as a movement toward maturity or, in other words, toward a depressive position, where dependency needs are acknowledged, as well as loving and negative feelings towards an attachment figure of loved one. Many adolescents will leave the treatment before this develops, but evidence that the adolescent is moving toward consolidation of personality structure is important in order for the adolescent and therapist to feel confident that it is the right time to start thinking of termination.

# Ending Treatment

From the beginning of the treatment process, we recognize that developmental features of adolescence and the demands of tolerating long-term treatment may be incompatible for some. These adolescents' need for immediate reward and their desire to demonstrate their autonomy and sense of independence from their parents may lead to resistance and a push to terminate the therapy process. In advising them and their parents, the therapist will need to assess the adolescent's motivation and try to distinguish between flight, with its risk for ongoing problems, and a move toward autonomy, with the implication of greater health and a movement in a positive developmental direction.

For the TFP-A therapist, the assessment involves an analysis of symptomatology and structural change. Because of resistances that could have come up during the course of treatment, it may have been necessary to review contract features at various times in order to remind the adolescent or parents of the goals and commitments all parties made and to ensure that the direction of treatment was not being lost. Doing this may have allowed for the recognition of progress that had been made as well as remaining areas of concern. Therefore, all participants should have some awareness of the relative progress made.

Structural change could be gauged in several ways:

1. Increased mentalization evidenced by the ability to reflect on problems and to no longer be characterized by an externalizing style that focused on what is wrong with parents, peers, and so forth. Continuing emotional growth requires adolescents to have a consistent, accurate perspective on themselves and others.
2. Decline in paranoid defenses, reflected in the transference and in the patient's report of relationships.
3. Decline in use of developmentally immature defenses such as splitting, idealization, or devaluation, and increase of representations of self and other that reflect greater integration of positive and negative attributes.
4. Improved work/school functioning, including improved performance based on increased ability to sustain effort, reduced procrastination, more consistent completion of assignments, and greater recognition of a need for assistance and willingness to obtain it.
5. Improved relationships with friends, including establishing closer friendships (e.g., having a "best friend" or boyfriend/girlfriend), having a more realistic and complex representation of others, and being less influenced by negative tendencies in others, including antisocial features.
6. Development of or improvement in sexual/loving relationships, including a movement from an egocentric orientation (e.g., "What's in it for me?"—enhanced status among others, personal pleasure only) toward a greater concern about the feelings of one's partner, as well as an ability to hold and acknowledge loving and hateful feelings toward important others.

Adolescents borderline PD who come for psychotherapy have varied treatment histories. For some, this may be their first experience, but others likely have a longer treatment history because borderline PD features may first appear in childhood, manifesting as impulsive, oppositional behaviors and mood and anxiety disorders. For those who would find extended treatment difficult, their safety from suicidal or other self-harming behaviors would be the major criterion to be met for stopping treatment. But for others whose condition has improved and who want to stop treatment, we advocate supporting them in this after a thorough discussion of the course of their treatment, their reasons for stopping, and their understanding of their gains and remaining issues to be worked through. Many adolescents with borderline or other PDs are likely to need additional psychotherapy at various other times in their life, including in young adulthood. It can be valuable for them to view psychotherapy not as a "life sentence" imposed on them by adults, in which they must continue to participate until they are old enough to break free, but as a helpful therapeutic space where they can enter and leave and feel comfortable about reentering in the future based on a felt internal need and personal decision.

Another group of patients bring up termination and complain to their parents about continuing therapy based on what is believed to be a resistance related to where they are in their treatment and to particular demands in their life. Active discussion and interpretation are in order so that they can reevaluate and better understand their use of avoidance. This group includes those who, despite the expected push for autonomy among adolescents, feel anxious about greater independence and movement toward adulthood and seek to maintain some semblance of the status quo. Others may feel more distraught as they delve further into the sources of their anxieties, including their aggressive and sexual underpinnings.

For those who are at an appropriate point for stopping treatment, termination can be done in a well-thought-out manner. A stopping time can be selected, and the therapy can work toward this termination date. Sadness may arise, as would occur with any interpersonal loss, and the original symptoms can reappear, in muted versions, and serve as a form of reminiscence. The process also includes an acknowledgment that the adolescent can return at a later time or see someone else in the future if the need arises. Throughout this process, there should be a genuine sense of accomplishment and pride and a recognition of the adolescent's successful effort, both individually and while working with someone in a relationship marked by cooperation and mutual concern.

# CHAPTER 9

# Conclusion

**IN THIS BOOK** we have introduced Transference-Focused Psychotherapy for Adolescents (TFP-A), a new treatment for adolescents with personality disorders, and have described its theoretical basis within an object relations and transference-focused model, as well as the treatment rationale and goal. We have outlined the tactics, strategies, and techniques used to help adolescents with personality disorders reduce the negative impacts during this crucial developmental period.

To summarize, TFP-A is a psychodynamic treatment for adolescents with borderline personality disorder delivered in individual sessions ideally twice a week but not less than once a week. The major goals of TFP-A are gaining a better behavioral control; increasing affect regulation; developing more intimate and gratifying relationships with family, peers, or close friends; and engaging in a productive life as well as investing in school and future goals. These goals can be met through the development of integrated representations of self and others, modification of primitive defense systems, resolution of identity diffusion that contributes to the fragmentation of the adolescent's internal world, and the safeguarding of every attempt made by the adolescent to face normal developmental challenges, which is often confounded or hijacked by the pathology itself. TFP-A comprises a series of tactics, strategies, and techniques geared toward achieving these goals.

We trust that we have succeeded in conveying a sense of what can be achieved using TFP-A. We hope that this will encourage clinicians to use an object relations and transference-focused approach as outlined in this book to help adolescents with personality disorders.

Looking back, we have built on the clinical and theoretical work done by Paulina Kernberg, a true pioneer who advocated for the early identification and treatment of personality disorders. As always, much remains to be done, but we hope to have inspired the next generation of clinicians to believe that effective treatment of adolescents with personality disorders is possible.

# APPENDIX

TFP-A Manual Adherence and
Competence Scale
(TFP-A/MACS)

# APPENDIX

# TFP-A Manual Adherence and Competence Scale (TFP-A/MACS)[1]

---

### SESSION DATA

| | |
|---|---|
| Therapist Name: | |
| Patient Initial–Subnum: | |
| Session Number: | Rater Name: |
| Session Date: | Date: |

## Introduction

The TFP-A Manual offers practical guidance for conducting psychotherapy sessions with adolescents who exhibit severe personality disorders. The TFP-A Manual facilitates standardization of the therapy method through an emphasis on adherence and competence in training of TFP-A therapists and of a clinical trial protocol. The goal of the TFP-A Manual Adherence and Competence Scale, hereafter referred to as TFP-A/MACS, is to outline procedures that establish and assess adherence to the TFP-A treatment manual and therapist competence in conducting TFP-A psychotherapy.

The TFP-A/MACS is a significant effort to guarantee the quality of outcome study data. By overseeing the implementation of the study methodology, the TFP-A developers are able to ensure that the application of treatment is as intended, which serves to enhance the quality of care for ad-

---

[1]Reprinted from Normandin L, Ensink K, Weiner A, et al.: *TFP-A Manual Adherence and Competence Scale*. Unpublished document, Laval University, 2017.

olescents and their parents, and also that the application of treatment is consistent, so that the developers can pool data across studies for conjoint analyses.

The TFP-A/MACS is fundamentally a data quality assurance and standardization process. By administering adherence ratings of therapy session videos, based on adherence and competence criteria, the developers aim to assure the overall quality of the treatment process.

# TFP-A/MACS Rater Qualifications

A typical TFP-A/MACS rater would be a *TFP-A certified supervisor* who is training TFP-A therapists prior to the beginning of the trial[2] or a *research assistant* who is willing to learn about TFP-A treatment or is in training to be a certified therapist. The following specifications are essential:

- Formal, graduate-level training and clinical skills in child and adolescent psychotherapy with a prerequisite of professional ethics in therapy
- Practicum, internship, or equivalent experience with direct patient contact in psychotherapy
- Openness to feedback
- Respect for the confidential nature of the video data
- Completion of TFP-A/MACS rater training

# Rating Adherence and Competence

For all items, supervisors or raters must distinguish between the TFP-A therapist's 1) *adherence*, which is the frequency and extensiveness of using specific TFP-A tactics or strategies, and 2) *competence*, which is the skill level of implementing those strategies. The specific system for coding the interview for adherence and competence is described in the following paragraphs.

---

[2]According to the International Society of Transference-Focused Psychotherapy (ISTFP) Training and Education Committee Levels of Certification in TFP-A, therapists who have achieved level C (i.e., certified TFP-A therapist) are eligible to participate in a research trial and to pursue ongoing TFP-A supervision with adherence and competence checks. The principal investigator (PI) is responsible for deciding what is a sufficient adherence and competence level according to the study design. The PI has to be approved by the ISTFP Research and Publication Committee.

# 1. Adherence: Frequency and Extensiveness

The adherence rating blends together both *frequency* (i.e., the number of discrete times the therapist engages in the intervention) and *extensiveness* (i.e., the depth or detail with which the therapist covers any given intervention) domains. These separate but related dimensions inform each rating interactively. In other words, the highest ratings involve a therapist's behaviors that are high in both frequency and extensiveness, whereas middle-range scores may reflect behaviors that were done less often or with less depth. All supervisors or raters use the following definitions to make their final rating for each item.[3]

| Rating | | |
|---|---|---|
| 1 | Not at all | The item never explicitly occurred. |
| 2 | A little | The item occurred once and was not addressed in any depth. |
| 3 | Infrequent | The item occurred twice but was not addressed in depth or detail. |
| 4 | Somewhat | The item occurred one time and in some detail, OR the item occurred three or four times, but all interventions were very brief. |
| 5 | Quite a bit | The item occurred more than once in the session and at least once in some detail or depth, OR the item occurred five or six times, but all interventions were very brief. |
| 6 | Considerably | The item occurred several times during the session and almost always with relative depth and detail, OR the item occurred more than six times, but all interventions were very brief. |
| 7 | Extensively | The item occurred many times, almost to the point of dominating the session, and was addressed in elaborate depth and detail, OR the item occurred briefly at such a high frequency that it became difficult to count. |

---

[3]In a subsequent version of the TFP-A/MACS, the guide will provide examples of therapist's adherent or competent behaviors that are rated on each item.

# 2. Competence: Skill Level

The therapist's competence or skill level refers to the therapist's demonstration of 1) expertise and competence, 2) appropriate timing of intervention, 3) clarity of language, and 4) responsiveness to where the patient (adolescent or parents) appears to be.

| Rating | | |
|---|---|---|
| 1 | Unsatisfactory | The therapist handles the item poorly (e.g., showing clear lack of expertise, understanding, competence, or commitment; inappropriate timing; unclear language). |
| 2 | Satisfactory | The therapist handles the item in an acceptable but less than "average" manner. |
| 3 | Good | The therapist handles the item in a manner characteristic of an "average," "good enough" therapist. |
| 4 | Very Good | The therapist demonstrates skill and expertise in handling the item. |
| 5 | Excellent | The therapist demonstrates a high level of excellence and mastery in this area. |

Although there may be significant overlap between therapist competence and effectiveness as measured by the adolescent's or parents' verbal response, competence is not the same as effectiveness, in the sense that it does not require the patient's positive response. Therefore, a therapist may score highly on competence for a particular item regardless of the patient's response.

Of equal importance, *competence* must be distinguished from *adherence*. For example, a therapist's score of "6" on frequency and extensiveness for a particular item does not necessarily mean the skill level was high. Supervisors or raters should rate competence independently of adherence. Thus, it is perfectly appropriate for a supervisor or a rater to give a rating of "3" on competence, even if the frequency and extensiveness rating is a "6."

# Phases of TFP-A

The TFP-A/MACS is divided into three sections corresponding to specific phases of the TFP-A treatment: A) assessment and contract setting, B) treatment implementation, and C) treatment interruption/termination.

## Section A: Adherence (Assessment and Contract) and Competence in Treatment Setting

These elements do not have to be accomplished in any specific order, nor will all of them likely be accomplished in one session. However, they must all be accomplished during the preliminary sessions (assessment and contract setting) that occur prior to implementing the treatment.

| # | Items | Adherence Rating[a] | | | | | | | | Competence Rating[b] | | | | | |
|---|---|---|---|---|---|---|---|---|---|---|---|---|---|---|---|
| | | N/A | 1 | 2 | 3 | 4 | 5 | 6 | 7 | N/A | 1 | 2 | 3 | 4 | 5 |
| 1 | Did the therapist demonstrate an appropriate level of engagement with the adolescent and/or parents? | | | | | | | | | | | | | | |
| 2 | Did the therapist explore: | | | | | | | | | | | | | | |
| | Identity confusion vs. diffusion ☐ | | | | | | | | | | | | | | |
| | Self-Other representations ☐ | | | | | | | | | | | | | | |
| | Primitive defenses ☐ | | | | | | | | | | | | | | |
| | Aggression ☐ | | | | | | | | | | | | | | |
| | Sexuality ☐ | | | | | | | | | | | | | | |
| | Reality testing ☐ | | | | | | | | | | | | | | |
| | Moral value system ☐ | | | | | | | | | | | | | | |
| | Academic/Work ☐ | | | | | | | | | | | | | | |
| | Level/Quality of mentalization ☐ | | | | | | | | | | | | | | |
| 3 | Did the therapist pay enough attention to the here-and-now interaction? | | | | | | | | | | | | | | |
| 4 | Did the therapist explore normal developmental issues (e.g., body change, separation from parents, career choice/future, romance)? | | | | | | | | | | | | | | |
| 5 | Did the therapist draw attention to the adolescent's behavior and interaction with the therapist? | | | | | | | | | | | | | | |

| # | Items | Adherence Rating[a] | | | | | | | | Competence Rating[b] | | | | | |
|---|---|---|---|---|---|---|---|---|---|---|---|---|---|---|---|
| | | N/A | 1 | 2 | 3 | 4 | 5 | 6 | 7 | N/A | 1 | 2 | 3 | 4 | 5 |
| 6 | Did the therapist pay adequate attention to the adolescent's goals/tasks in therapy and parents' expectancies/level of participation? | | | | | | | | | | | | | | |
| 7 | Was the therapist able to help the adolescent to recognize the need for treatment and help him/her to define treatment priorities? | | | | | | | | | | | | | | |
| 8 | Did the therapist assess specific threats to the treatment (adolescent and parents)? | | | | | | | | | | | | | | |
| 9 | Did the therapist offer the adolescent and parents an understanding of symptoms and dysfunctions as being based in an underlying personality disorder? | | | | | | | | | | | | | | |
| 10 | Did the therapist define the responsibilities of the adolescent and those of the parents? | | | | | | | | | | | | | | |
| 11 | Did the therapist detail the "least restrictive" set of conditions necessary to ensure the treatment to unfold? | | | | | | | | | | | | | | |
| 12 | Did the therapist establish specific parameters to limit the threats to the treatment or secondary gains? | | | | | | | | | | | | | | |
| 13 | Did the therapist confront the parent's threats to the treatment? | | | | | | | | | | | | | | |
| 14 | Overall, did the therapist create conditions in which psychodynamic exploration can take place, i.e., feel comfortable and safe enough to remain neutral and think clearly? | | | | | | | | | | | | | | |

[a]Adherence: 1 = not at all; 2 = a little; 3 = infrequent; 4 = somewhat; 5 = quite a bit; 6 = considerably; 7 = extensively.
[b]Competence: 1 = unsatisfactory; 2 = satisfactory; 3 = good; 4 = very good; 5 = excellent.

**Explanation of "Not at All" Adherence and "Unsatisfactory" Competence**

_____
_____
_____
_____
_____
_____
_____
_____
_____
_____
_____
_____
_____
_____
_____
_____
_____
_____
_____
_____
_____
_____
_____
_____
_____
_____
_____

# Section B: Adherence and Competence in Treatment Implementation

These elements do not have to be accomplished in any specific order, nor will all of them likely be accomplished in one session. However, they must all be accomplished during the overall duration of the treatment.

| # | Items | Adherence Rating[a] | | | | | | | | Competence Rating[b] | | | | | |
|---|---|---|---|---|---|---|---|---|---|---|---|---|---|---|---|
| | | N/A | 1 | 2 | 3 | 4 | 5 | 6 | 7 | N/A | 1 | 2 | 3 | 4 | 5 |
| 1 | Did the therapist demonstrate an appropriate level of engagement with the adolescent? | | | | | | | | | | | | | | |
| 2 | Was the therapist able to clearly define/maintain the implication of the parent's behavior without interfering with the adolescent's work? | | | | | | | | | | | | | | |
| 3 | Did the therapist demonstrate flexibility in using tactics? | | | | | | | | | | | | | | |
| 4 | Did the therapist attend to the frame/contract if there are relevant issues or emergency priorities? | | | | | | | | | | | | | | |
| 5 | Did the therapist maintain neutrality? | | | | | | | | | | | | | | |
| 6 | Did the therapist give guideline to the adolescent on how to explore internal world (mentalization)? | | | | | | | | | | | | | | |
| 7 | Did the therapist use clarification? | | | | | | | | | | | | | | |
| 8 | Did the therapist use confrontation? | | | | | | | | | | | | | | |
| 9 | Did the therapist interpret clearly and understandingly the adolescent's: | | | | | | | | | | | | | | |
| | Acting out □ | | | | | | | | | | | | | | |
| | Somatization □ | | | | | | | | | | | | | | |
| | Developmental regression □ | | | | | | | | | | | | | | |
| | Resistance to transference □ | | | | | | | | | | | | | | |
| | Conflict □ | | | | | | | | | | | | | | |

| # | Items | Adherence Rating[a] | | | | | | | | Competence Rating[b] | | | | | |
|---|-------|:-:|:-:|:-:|:-:|:-:|:-:|:-:|:-:|:-:|:-:|:-:|:-:|:-:|:-:|
| | | N/A | 1 | 2 | 3 | 4 | 5 | 6 | 7 | N/A | 1 | 2 | 3 | 4 | 5 |
| 10 | Did the therapist identify the proper activated transference? | | | | | | | | | | | | | | |
| | Paranoid transference ☐ | | | | | | | | | | | | | | |
| | Narcissistic transference ☐ | | | | | | | | | | | | | | |
| | Psychopathic transference ☐ | | | | | | | | | | | | | | |
| | Depressive transference ☐ | | | | | | | | | | | | | | |
| 11 | Did the therapist pay adequate attention to developments in external reality related to developments in the session and vice versa? | | | | | | | | | | | | | | |
| 12 | Did the therapist attend to enactments embedded in the patient's verbal and non-verbal communication? | | | | | | | | | | | | | | |
| 13 | Did the therapist bring to the adolescent's awareness a clear affectively dominant issue in the session? | | | | | | | | | | | | | | |
| 14 | Did the therapist call attention to the dominant self-object dyad related to the affectively dominant issue? | | | | | | | | | | | | | | |
| | In the transference ☐ | | | | | | | | | | | | | | |
| | In the extratransferential ☐ | | | | | | | | | | | | | | |
| 15 | Did the therapist offer interpretation with the aim of integrating split-off transferences with their opposite counterparts? | | | | | | | | | | | | | | |

| # | Items | Adherence Rating[a] | | | | | | | | Competence Rating[b] | | | | | |
|---|---|---|---|---|---|---|---|---|---|---|---|---|---|---|---|
| | | N/A | 1 | 2 | 3 | 4 | 5 | 6 | 7 | N/A | 1 | 2 | 3 | 4 | 5 |
| 16 | Did it appear that countertransference interfered with the therapist's attitude or interventions in the session? | | | | | | | | | | | | | | |
| 17 | Did the therapist pay adequate attention to the treatment goals and keep the "big picture" in mind? | | | | | | | | | | | | | | |
| 18 | Overall, was the therapist able to create conditions in which elaboration of the adolescent's internal world took place confidentially and safely while maintaining an appropriate level of the parent's collaboration? | | | | | | | | | | | | | | |

[a]Adherence: 1=not at all; 2=a little; 3=infrequent; 4=somewhat; 5=quite a bit; 6=considerably; 7=extensively.
[b]Competence: 1=unsatisfactory; 2=satisfactory; 3=good; 4=very good; 5=excellent.

Adolescent's response to interventions

1. Patient rejected the therapist's interventions most of the time. ☐

2. Patient ignored the therapist's interventions most of the time. ☐

3. Patient accepted superficially the therapist's interventions most of the time. ☐

4. Patient responded to therapist's interventions with thoughtfulness most of the time. ☐

5. Patient responded to therapist's interventions with thoughtfulness and further exploration most of the time. ☐

Therapist's response to patient's response

1. Therapist did not explore the patient's response to intervention most of the time. ☐

2. Therapist briefly noted patient's response, but did not explore most of the time. ☐

3. Therapist described the patient's response, but did not explore further most of the time. ☐

4. Therapist described the patient's response and briefly explored most of the time. ☐

5. Therapist described the patient's response and linked it to the dominant theme in some depth most of the time. ☐

Therapist's response to previous supervision

Did the therapist learn from the previous supervision?     Yes ☐ No ☐

## Explanation of "Not at All" Adherence and "Unsatisfactory" Competence

_____

_____

_____

_____

_____

_____

# Section C: Adherence and Competence in Treatment Interruption/Termination

| # | Items | Adherence Rating[a] | | | | | | | | Competence Rating[b] | | | | | |
|---|-------|-----|---|---|---|---|---|---|---|-----|---|---|---|---|---|
| | | N/A | 1 | 2 | 3 | 4 | 5 | 6 | 7 | N/A | 1 | 2 | 3 | 4 | 5 |
| 1 | In case of premature termination, was the therapist able to confront the adolescent and parents? | | | | | | | | | | | | | | |
| 2 | Did the therapist negotiate a "temporary interruption" of the treatment? | | | | | | | | | | | | | | |
| 3 | Was the therapist able to identify "negative therapeutic reactions" indicative of the adolescent's improvement? | | | | | | | | | | | | | | |
| 4 | Was the therapist able to recognize the adolescent's experience of mixed or negative feelings prior to termination, echoing past losses and hurts and often accompanied by a return of their primary symptoms and behaviors? | | | | | | | | | | | | | | |
| 5 | Was the therapist able to explore and analyze the underlying unconscious feelings toward separation/termination: | | | | | | | | | | | | | | |
| | Sadness-Gratitude /Normal reaction ☐ | | | | | | | | | | | | | | |
| | Guilt/Neurotic depressive reaction ☐ | | | | | | | | | | | | | | |
| | Rage/Borderline reaction ☐ | | | | | | | | | | | | | | |
| | Indifference/Narcissistic reaction ☐ | | | | | | | | | | | | | | |
| | Triumph/Psychopathic reaction ☐ | | | | | | | | | | | | | | |
| 6 | Did it appear that countertransference interfered with the therapist's working on terminating the treatment? | | | | | | | | | | | | | | |

[a] Adherence: 1 = not at all; 2 = a little; 3 = infrequent; 4 = somewhat; 5 = quite a bit; 6 = considerably; 7 = extensively.
[b] Competence: 1 = unsatisfactory; 2 = satisfactory; 3 = good; 4 = very good; 5 = excellent.

## Treatment termination (last session)

Did the adolescent show an improvement in

Symptoms ☐

Behaviors ☐

Interpersonal relationships ☐

Mentalization ☐

Personality organization ☐

Did the parents acknowledge the adolescent's change?

Yes ☐    No ☐    Somewhat ☐

Has there been a resumption of development (toward normal development)?

Yes ☐    No ☐    Somewhat ☐

# Explanation of "Not at All" Adherence and "Unsatisfactory" Competence

_____

_____

_____

_____

_____

_____

_____

_____

_____

_____

_____

_____

_____

_____

_____

_____

_____

# References

Achenbach TM: Applications of the Achenbach System of Empirically Based Assessment (ASEBA) to children, adolescents, and their parents, in The Clinical Assessment of Children and Adolescents: A Practitioners' Guide. Edited by Smith SR, Handler L. Mahwah, NJ, Erlbaum, 2006, pp 329–346

Afifi TO, Mather A, Boman J, et al: Childhood adversity and personality disorders: results from a nationally representative population-based study. J Psychiatr Res 45(6):814–822, 2011

Akhtar S, Samuel S: The concept of identity: developmental origins, phenomenology, clinical relevance, and measurement. Harv Rev Psychiatry 3(5):254–267, 1996

Amad A, Ramoz N, Thomas P, et al: Genetics of borderline personality disorder: systematic review and proposal of an integrative model. Neurosci Biobehav Rev 40:6–19, 2014

American Psychiatric Association: Diagnostic and Statistical Manual of Mental Disorders, 5th Edition. Arlington, VA, American Psychiatric Association, 2013

Arens EA, Stopsack M, Spitzer C, et al: Borderline personality disorder in four different age groups: a cross-sectional study of community residents in Germany. J Pers Disord 27(2):196–207, 2013

Auchincloss EL, Samberg E: Psychoanalytic Terms and Concepts, 4th Edition. Washington, DC, American Psychoanalytic Association, 2012

Barkley RA: Barkley Deficits in Executive Functioning Scale—Children and Adolescents (BDEFS-CA). New York, Guilford, 2012

Battle CL, Shea MT, Johnson DM, et al: Childhood maltreatment associated with adult personality disorders: findings from the Collaborative Longitudinal Personality Disorders Study. J Pers Disord 18(2):193–211, 2004

Beck JS, Beck AT, Jolly JB: Beck Youth Inventories, 2nd Edition. San Antonio, TX, Pearson Assessments, 2005

Becker DF, Grilo CM, Edell WS, et al: Diagnostic efficiency of borderline personality disorder criteria in hospitalized adolescents: comparison with hospitalized adults. Am J Psychiatry 159(12):2042–2047, 2002

Beebe B: Mother-infant mutual influence and precursors of self- and object representations, in Empirical Studies of Psychoanalytic Studies, Vol 2. Edited by Masling J. Hillsdale, NJ, Analytic Press, 1986, pp 27–48).

Bégin M, Ensink K, Chabot S, et al: Childhood maltreatment, adolescent psychological difficulties and borderline personality features: a personcentered approach. Adolescent Psychiatry 7(4):330–343, 2017

Belsky DW, Caspi A, Arseneault L, et al: Etiological features of borderline personality related characteristics in a birth cohort of 12-year-old children. Dev Psychopathol 24(1):251–265, 2012

Biberdzic M, Ensink K, Normandin L, Clarkin JF: Empirical typology of adolescent personality organization. J Adolesc 66:31–48, 2018

Birkeland MS, Melkevik O, Holsen I, et al: Trajectories of global self-esteem development during adolescence. J Adolesc 35(1):43–54, 2012

Blos P: Intensive psychotherapy in relation to the various phases of the adolescent period. Am J Orthopsychiatry 32(5):901–910, 1962

Bornovalova MA, Hicks BM, Iacono WG, et al: Stability, change, and heritability of borderline personality disorder traits from adolescence to adulthood: a longitudinal twin study. Dev Psychopathol 21(4):1335–1353, 2009

Bounoua N, Felton JF, Long K, et al: Childhood emotional abuse and borderline personality features: the role of anxiety sensitivity among adolescents. Personal Ment Health 9(2):87–95, 2015

Brummelman E, Thomaes S, Nelemans SA, et al: Origins of narcissism in children. Proc Natl Acad Sci U S A 112(12):3659–3662, 2015

Caligor E, Kernberg OF, Clarkin JF: Handbook of Dynamic Psychotherapy for Higher Level Personality Pathology. Washington, DC, American Psychiatric Publishing, 2007

Caligor E, Kernberg OF, Clarkin JF, et al: Psychodynamic Therapy for Personality Pathology: Treating Self and Interpersonal Functioning. Washington, DC, American Psychiatric Association Publishing, 2018

Campbell WK, Miller JD: The Handbook of Narcissism and Narcissistic Personality Disorder: Theoretical Approaches, Empirical Findings, and Treatments. Hoboken, NJ, Wiley, 2011

Carlson EA, Egeland B, Sroufe LA: A prospective investigation of the development of borderline personality symptoms. Dev Psychopathol 21(4):1311–1334, 2009

Carriedo N, Corral A, Montoro PR, et al: The development of metaphor comprehension and its relationship with relational verbal reasoning and executive function. PLoS One 11(3):e0150289, 2016

Case R, Okamoto Y: The role of central conceptual structures in the development of children's thought. Monogr Soc Res Child Dev 61(1–2):v–265.10.2307/1166077, 1996

Casey BJ: Beyond simple models of self-control to circuit-based accounts of adolescent behavior. Annu Rev Psychol 66:295–319, 2015

Casey BJ, Jones RM: Neurobiology of the adolescent brain and behavior. J Am Acad Child Adolesc Psychiatry 49(12):1189–1285, 2010

Chabrol H, Montovany A, Chouicha K, et al: Frequency of borderline personality disorder in a sample of French high school students. Can J Psychiatry 46(9):847–849, 2001

Chanen AM, Kaess M: Developmental pathways to borderline personality disorder. Current Psychiatry Rep 14(1):45–53, 2012

Chanen AM, McCutcheon LK: Personality disorder in adolescence: the diagnosis that dare not speak its name. Personal Ment Health 2(1):35–41, 2008

Chanen AM, McCutcheon L: Prevention and early intervention for borderline personality disorder: current status and recent evidence. Br J Psychiatry 54(suppl):s24–s29, 2013

Chanen AM, Jackson HJ, McGorry PD, et al: Two-year stability of personality disorder in older adolescent outpatients. J Pers Disord 18(6):526–541, 2004

Chanen AM, Jovev M, Jackson HJ: Adaptive functioning and psychiatric symptoms in adolescents with borderline personality disorder. J Clin Psychiatry 68:297–306, 2007

Chiesa M, Fonagy P: Reflective function as a mediator between childhood adversity, personality disorder and symptom distress. Personal Ment Health 8(1):52–66, 2014

Cicchetti D, Rogosch FA: A developmental psychopathology perspective on adolescence. J Consult Clin Psychol 70(1):6–20, 2002

Cicchetti D, Toth SL: Child maltreatment and developmental psychopathology: a multilevel perspective. in Developmental Psychopathology, Vol 3: Maladaptation and Psychopathology. Edited by Cicchetti D. Hoboken, NJ, Wiley, 2016, pp 1–55

Cicchetti D, Valentino K: An ecological-transactional perspective on child maltreatment: failure of the average expectable environment and its influence on child development, in Developmental Psychopathology: Risk, Disorder, and Adaptation. Edited by Cicchetti D, Cohen DJ. Hoboken, NJ, Wiley, 2006, pp 129–201

Clarkin JF, Posner M: Defining the mechanisms of borderline personality disorder. Psychopathology 38(2):56–63, 2005

Clarkin JF, Yeomans FE, Kernberg OF: Psychotherapy for Borderline Personality: Focusing on Object Relations. Washington, DC, American Psychiatric Publishing, 2006

Clarkin JF, Levy KN, Lenzenweger MF, et al: Evaluating three treatments for borderline personality disorder: a multiwave study. Am J Psychiatry 164(4):922–928, 2007

Coghill D: Editorial: Acknowledging complexity and heterogeneity in causality—implications of recent insights into neuropsychology of childhood disorders for clinical practice. J Child Psychol Psychiatry 55(7):737–740, 2014

Cohen P, Crawford TN, Johnson JG, et al: The Children in the Community Study of developmental course of personality disorder. J Pers Disord 19(5):466–486, 2005

Cohen P, Chen H, Crawford TN, et al: Personality disorders in early adolescence and the development of later substance use disorders in the general population. Drug Alcohol Depend 88 (suppl 1):71–84, 2007

Conners KC: Conners, 3rd Edition (Conners 3). Toronto, Ontario, Canada, Multi-Health Systems, 2008

Crawford TN, Cohen P, First MB, et al: Comorbid Axis I and Axis II disorders in early adolescence: outcomes 20 years later. Arch Gen Psychiatry 65(6):641–648, 2008

Crocetti E, Branje S, Rubini M, et al: Identity processes and parent-child and sibling relationships in adolescence: a five-wave multi-informant longitudinal study. Child Dev 88(1):210–228, 2017

Cross D, Fani N, Powers A, et al: Neurobiological development in the context of childhood trauma. Clin Psychol (New York) 24(2):111–124, 2017

Crowe ML, LoPilato AC, Campbell WK, et al: Identifying two groups of entitled individuals: cluster analysis reveals emotional stability and self-esteem distinction. J Pers Disord 30(6):762–775, 2016

Crowell SE, Beauchaine TP, Linehan MM: A biosocial developmental model of borderline personality: elaborating and extending Linehan's theory. Psychol Bull 135(3):495–510, 2009

Crowell SE, Kaufman EA, Beauchaine TP: A biosocial model of BPD: theory and empirical evidence, in Handbook of Borderline Personality Disorder in Children and Adolescents. Edited by Sharp C, Tackett JL. New York, Springer Science+Business Media, 2014, pp 143–157

Damasio AR: Brain and language: what a difference a decade makes. Curr Opin Neurology 10(3):177–178, 1994a

Damasio AR: Descartes' Error: Emotion, Reason, and the Human Brain. New York, Grosset/Putnam, 1994b

De Clercq B, Decuyper M, De Caluwé E: Developmental manifestations of borderline personality pathology from an age-specific dimensional personality disorder trait framework, in Handbook of Borderline Personality Disorder in Children and Adolescents. Edited by Sharp C, Tackett J. New York, Science+Business Media, 2014, pp 81–94

DeFife JA, Malone JC, DiLallo J, et al: Assessing adolescent personality disorders with the Shedler–Westen Assessment Procedure for Adolescents. Clin Psychol (New York) 20(4):393–407, 2013

Diamond D, Yeomans FE, Levy K: Psychodynamic psychotherapy for narcissistic personality disorder, in The Handbook of Narcissism and Narcissistic Personality Disorder: Theoretical Approaches, Empirical Findings, and Treatment. Edited by Campbell K, Miller J. New York, Wiley, 2011, pp 423–433

Dickinson KA, Pincus AL: Interpersonal analysis of grandiose and vulnerable narcissism. J Pers Disord 17(3):188–207, 2003

Distel MA, Hottenga J-J, Trull TJ, et al: Chromosome 9: linkage for borderline personality disorder features. Psychiatr Genet 18(6):302–307, 2008

Doering S, Hörz S, Rentrop M, et al: Transference-focused psychotherapy v. treatment by community psychotherapists for borderline personality disorder: randomised controlled trial. Br J Psychiatry 196(5):389–395, 2010

Elkind D: Egocentrism in adolescence. Child Dev 38(4):1025–1034, 1967

Epstein S: Integration of the cognitive and the psychodynamic unconscious. Am Psychol 49(8):709–724, 1994

Erikson EH: Childhood and Society. New York, Norton, 1950

Erikson EH: Identity: Youth and Crisis. New York, Norton, 1968

Evans JStBT: Dual-processing accounts of reasoning, judgment, and social cognition. Annu Rev Psychol 59(1):255–278, 2008

Evans JStBT, Handley SJ, Over DE, Perham N: Background beliefs in Bayesian inference. Mem Cognit 30(2):179–190, 2002

Fairbairn WRD: Psychoanalytic Studies of the Personality. London, Routledge & Kegan Paul, 1952

Feenstra DJ, Busschbach JJV, Verheul R, et al: Prevalence and comorbidity of Axis I and Axis II disorders among treatment refractory adolescents admitted for specialized psychotherapy. J Pers Disord 25(6):842–850, 2011

Fonagy P, Gergely G, Jurist EL, et al: Affect Regulation, Mentalization, and the Development of the Self. New York, Other Press, 2002

Fossati A: Borderline personality disorder in adolescence: phenomenology and construct validity, in Handbook of Borderline Personality Disorder in Children and Adolescents. Edited by Sharp C, Tackett JL. New York, Springer Science+Business Media, 2014, pp 19–34

Frankel-Waldheter M, Macfie J, Strimpfel JM, et al: Effect of maternal autonomy and relatedness and borderline personality disorder on adolescent symptomatology. Personal Disord 6(2):152–160, 2015

Freud A: Adolescence. Psychoanal Study Child 13:255–278, 1958

Fruzzetti AE, Shenk C, Hoffman PD: Family interaction and the development of borderline personality disorder: a transactional model. Dev Psychopathol 17(4):1007–1030, 2005

Galvan A: Risky behavior in adolescents: the role of the developing brain, in The Adolescent Brain: Learning, Reasoning, and Decision Making. Edited by Reyna VF, Chapman SB, Dougherty MR, Confrey J. Washington, DC, American Psychological Association, 2012

Garland AF, Lewczyk-Boxmeyer CM, Gabayan EN, et al: Multiple stakeholder agreement on desired outcomes for adolescents' mental health services. Psychiatr Serv 55(6):671–676, 2004

Garnet KE, Levy KN, Mattanah JJ, et al: Borderline personality disorder in adolescents: ubiquitous or specific? Am J Psychiatry 151(9):1380–1382, 1994

Glenn CR, Klonsky ED: Prospective prediction of nonsuicidal self-injury: a 1-year longitudinal study in young adults. Behav Ther 42(4):751–762, 2011

Glenn CR, Klonsky ED: Reliability and validity of borderline personality disorder in hospitalized adolescents. J Can Acad Child Adolesc Psychiatry 22(3):206–211, 2013

Goodman M, New A, Siever L: Trauma, genes, and the neurobiology of personality disorders. Ann NY Acad Sci 1032:104–116, 2004

Griffiths M: Validity, utility and acceptability of borderline personality disorder diagnosis in childhood and adolescence: survey of psychiatrists. The Psychiatrist 35(1):19–22, 2011

Grilo CM, Becker DF, Fehon DC, et al: Gender differences in personality disorders in psychiatrically hospitalized adolescents. Am J Psychiatry 153(8):1089–1091, 1996

Gunderson JG, Stout RL, McGlashan TH, et al: Ten-year course of borderline personality disorder: psychopathology and function from the Collaborative Longitudinal Personality Disorders Study. Arch Gen Psychiatry 68(8):827–837, 2011

Guttman HA, Laporte L: Empathy in families of women with borderline personality disorder, anorexia nervosa, and a control group. Family Process 39(3):345–358, 2000

Ha C, Balderas JC, Zanarini MC, et al: Psychiatric comorbidity in hospitalized adolescents with borderline personality disorder. J Clin Psychiatry 75(5):e457–e464, 2014

Halford GS, Andrews G: Reasoning and problem solving, in Handbook of Child Psychology: Cognition, Perception, and Language, Vol 2, 6th Edition. Edited by Kuhn D, Siegler RS, Damon W, et al. Hoboken, NJ, Wiley, 2006, pp 557–608

Hammad TA, Laughren T, Racoosin J: Suicidality in pediatric patients treated with antidepressant drugs. Arch Gen Psychiatry 63(3):332–339, 2006

Harter S: The developing self, in Child and Adolescent Development: An Advanced Course. Edited by Damon W, Learner RM. Hoboken, NJ, Wiley, 2008, pp 216–262

Harter S: Emerging self-processes during childhood and adolescence, in Handbook of Self and Identity. Edited by Leary MR, Tangney JP. New York, Guilford, 2012, pp 680–715

Hawley KM, Weisz JR: Youth versus parent working alliance in usual clinical care: distinctive associations with retention, satisfaction, and treatment outcome. J Clin Child Adolesc Psychol 34(1):117–128, 2005

Haxhe S: Parentification and related processes: distinction and implications for clinical practice. Journal of Family Psychotherapy 27(3):185–199, 2016

Hutsebaut J, Feenstra DJ, Luyten P: Personality disorders in adolescence: label or opportunity? Clin Psychol (New York) 20(4):445–451, 2013

Jacobson AM, Beardslee W, Hauser ST, et al: Evaluating ego defense mechanisms using clinical interviews: an empirical study of adolescent diabetic and psychiatric patients. J Adolesc 9(4):303–319, 1986

Jacobson E: The Self and the Object World. Madison, CT, International Universities Press, 1964

Johnson JG, First MB, Cohen P, et al: Adverse outcomes associated with personality disorder not otherwise specified in a community sample. Am J Psychiatry 162(10):1926–1932, 2005

Johnson JG, Bromley E, Bornstein RF, et al: Adolescent personality disorders, in Behavioral and Emotional Disorders in Children and Adolescents: Nature, Assessment, and Treatment. Edited by Wolfe DA, Mash EJ. New York, Guilford, 2006, pp 463–484

Johnson JG, Cohen P, Kasen S, et al: Cumulative prevalence of personality disorders between adolescence and adulthood. Acta Psychiatr Scand 118(5):410–413, 2008

Jones RA, Wells M: An empirical study of parentification and personality. American Journal of Family Therapy 24(2):145–152, 1996

Jørgensen CR: Invited essay: Identity and borderline personality disorder. J Pers Disord 24:344–364, 2010

Jovev M, McKenzie T, Whittle S, et al: Temperament and maltreatment in the emergence of borderline and antisocial personality pathology during early adolescence. J Can Acad Child Adolesc Psychiatry 22(3):220–229, 2013

Joyce PR, McKenzie JM, Luty SE, et al: Temperament, childhood environment and psychopathology as risk factors for avoidant and borderline personality disorders. Aust N Z J Psychiatry 37(6):756–764, 2003

Kaufman J, Birmaher B, Brent D, et al: Schedule for Affective Disorders and Schizophrenia for School-Age Children—Present and Lifetime version (K-SADS-PL): initial reliability and validity data. J Am Acad Child Adolesc Psychiatry 36(7):980–988, 1997

Kendall T, Pilling S, Tyrer P: Borderline and antisocial personality disorder: summary of NICE guideline. BMJ 338:b93, 2009

Kernberg OF: Severe Personality Disorders. New Haven, CT, Yale University Press, 1984

Kernberg OF: Severe Personality Disorders: Psychotherapeutic Strategies. New Haven, CT, Yale University Press, 1993

Kernberg OF: Identity: recent findings and clinical implications, in The Inseparable Nature of Love and Aggression: Clinical and Theoretical Perspectives. Washington, DC, American Psychiatric Publishing, 2012, pp 3–30

Kernberg OF: Neurobiological correlates of object relations theory: the relationship between neurobiological and psychodynamic development. International Forum of Psychoanalysis 24(1):38–46, 2015

Kernberg OF: New developments in transference focused psychotherapy. Int J Psychoanal 97(2):385–407, 2016

Kernberg PF: Psychological interventions for the suicidal adolescent. Am J Psychother 48(1):52–63, 1994

Kernberg PF: Personality disorders in childhood and adolescent: an overview, in Handbook of Child and Adolescent Psychiatry, The Grade-School Child: Development and Syndromes. Edited by Kernberg PF, Bemporad JR. New York, Wiley, 1997, pp 610–622

Kernberg PF, Clarkin AJ, Greenblatt E, et al: The Cornell Interview of Peers and Friends: development and validation. J Am Acad Child Adolesc Psychiatry 31(3):483–489, 1992

Kernberg PF, Hajal F, Normandin L: Narcissistic personality disorder in adolescent inpatients: a retrospective record review study of descriptive characteristics, in Disorders of Narcissism: Diagnostic, Clinical, and Empirical Implications. Edited by Ronningstam EF. Washington, DC, American Psychiatric Association, 1998, pp 437–456

Kernberg PF, Weiner AS, Bardenstein KK: Personality Disorders in Children and Adolescents. New York, Basic Books, 2000

Khoury JE, Pechtel P, Andersen CM, et al: Relations among maternal withdrawal in infancy, borderline features, suicidality/self-injury, and adult hippocampal volume: a 30-year longitudinal study. Behav Brain Res 374:112139, 2019

King-Casas B, Sharp C, Lomax-Bream L, et al: The rupture and repair of cooperation in borderline personality disorder. Science 321(5890):806–810, 2008

Klein M: Mourning and its relation to manic-depressive states. Int J Psychoanal 21:125–153, 1940

Koenigsberg HW, Siever LJ, Lee H, et al: Neural correlates of emotion processing in borderline personality disorder. Psychiatry Res 172(3):192–199, 2009

Kohlberg L, Kramer R: Continuities and discontinuities in childhood and adult development. Hum Dev 12(2):3–120, 1969

Kroger J, Marcia JE: The identity statuses: origins, meanings, and interpretations, in Handbook of Identity Theory and Research, Vol 1. Edited by Schwartz SJ, Luyckx K, Vignoles VL. New York, Springer, 2011, pp 31–53

Kroger J, Martinussen M, Marcia JE: Identity status change during adolescence and young adulthood: a meta-analysis. J Adolesc 33:683–698, 2010

Kuhn D, Franklin S: The second decade: what develops (and how), in Handbook of Child Psychology: Cognition, Perception, and Language, Vol 2, 6th Edition. Edited by Kuhn D, Siegler RS, Damon W, et al. Hoboken, NJ, Wiley, 2006, pp 953–993

Laurenssen EMP, Hutsebaut J, Feenstra DJ, et al: Diagnosis of personality disorders in adolescents: a study among psychologists. Child Adolesc Psychiatry Ment Health 7(1):3, 2013

Lemery-Chalfant K, Clifford S, McDonald K, et al: Arizona Twin Project: a focus on early resilience. Twin Res Hum Genet 16(1):404–411, 2013a

Lemery-Chalfant K, Kao K, Swann G, et al: Childhood temperament: passive gene-environment correlation, gene-environment interaction, and the hidden importance of the family environment. Dev Psychopathol 25(1):51–63, 2013b

Lenzenweger MF, Cicchetti D: Toward a developmental psychopathology approach to borderline personality disorder. Dev Psychopathol 17(4):893–898, 2005

Lerner JS, Keltner D: Beyond valence: toward a model of emotion-specific influences on judgement and choice. Cognition and Emotion 14(4):473–493, 2000

Levy KN: The implications of attachment theory and research for understanding borderline personality disorder. Dev Psychopathol 17(4):959–986, 2005

Levy KN, Becker DF, Grilo CM, et al: Concurrent and predictive validity of the personality disorder diagnosis in adolescent patients. Am J Psychiatry 156(10):1522–1528, 1999

Lewinsohn PM, Rohde P, Seeley JR, et al: Axis II psychopathology as a function of Axis I disorders in childhood and adolescence. J Am Acad Child Adolesc Psychiatry 36(12):1752–1759, 1997

Lieberman MD: Introversion and working memory: central executive differences. Personality and Individual Differences 28(3):479–486, 2000

Livesley WJ: Behavioral and molecular genetic contributions to a dimensional classification of personality disorder. J Pers Disord 19(2):131–155, 2005

Livson N, Peskin H: Prediction of adult psychological health in a longitudinal study. J Abnorm Psychol 72(6):509–518, 1967

Loewenstein GF, Weber EU, Hsee CK, et al: Risk as feelings. Psychol Bull 127(2):267–286, 2001

Lyons-Ruth K: The two-person unconscious: intersubjective dialogue, enactive relational representation, and the emergence of new forms of relational organization. Psychoanalytic Inquiry 19(4):576–617, 1999

Lyons-Ruth K, Holmes BM, Sasvari-Szekely M, et al: Serotonin transporter polymorphism and borderline or antisocial traits among low-income young adults. Psychiatr Genet 17(6):339–343, 2007

Lyons-Ruth K, Bureau J-F, Easterbrooks M, et al: Parsing the construct of maternal insensitivity: distinct longitudinal pathways associated with early maternal withdrawal. Attach Hum Dev 15(5–6):562–582, 2013

Mahler MS: On the first three subphases of the separation-individuation process. Int J Psychoanal 53 (Pt 3):333–338, 1972a

Mahler MS: Rapprochement subphase of the separation-individuation process. Psychoanal Q 41(4):487–506, 1972b

Marcia JE, Archer SL: The Identity Status Interview, Late Adolescent College Form, in Ego Identity: A Handbook for Psychosocial Research. Edited by Marcia JE, Waterman AS, Matteson DR, et al. New York, Springer-Verlag, 1993, pp 205–240

McManus M, Lerner HD, Robbins D, et al: Assessment of borderline symptomatology in hospitalized adolescents. J Am Acad Child Psychiatry 23(6):685–694, 1984

Meares R, Gerull F, Stevenson J, et al: Is self disturbance the core of borderline personality disorder? An outcome study of borderline personality factors. Aust N Z J Psychiatry 45(3):214–222, 2011

Mechanic KL, Barry CT: Adolescent grandiose and vulnerable narcissism: associations with perceived parenting practices. Journal of Child and Family Studies 24(5):1510–1518, 2015

Meijer M, Goedhart AW, Treffers PDA: The persistence of borderline personality disorder in adolescence. J Pers Disord 12(1):13–22, 1998

Michonski JD: The underlying factor structure of DSM criteria in youth BPD, in Handbook of Borderline Personality Disorder in Children and Adolescents. Edited by Sharp C, Tackett JL. New York, Springer Science & Business Media, 2014, pp 35–48

Michonski JD, Sharp C, Steinberg L, et al: An item response theory analysis of the DSM-IV borderline personality disorder criteria in a population-based sample of 11- to 12-year-old children. Personal Disord 4(1):15–22, 2013

Miller AL, Muehlenkamp JJ, Jacobson CM: Fact or fiction: diagnosing borderline personality disorder in adolescents. Clin Psychol Rev 28(6):969–981, 2008

Moffitt TE: Adolescence-limited and life-course-persistent antisocial behavior: a developmental taxonomy. Psychol Rev 100(4):674–701, 1993a

Moffitt TE: The neuropsychology of conduct disorder. Dev Psychopathol 5(1–2):135–151, 1993b

National Health and Medical Research Council: Clinical Practice Guideline for the Management of Borderline Personality Disorder. Melbourne, Australia, National Health and Medical Research Council, 2012

National Institute for Clinical Excellence: Borderline personality disorder: treatment and management. Clinical Guideline 78. 2009. London, National Collaborating Centre for Mental Health. Available at: www.guidance.nice.org.uk/CG78. Accessed May 27, 2020.

Oldham JM: DSM models of personality disorders. Curr Opin Psychol 2:86–88, 2018

Panksepp J, Biven L: The Norton Series on Interpersonal Neurobiology. The Archaeology of Mind: Neuroevolutionary Origins of Human Emotion. New York, WW Norton, 2012

Paris J: Personality Disorders Over Time. Washington, DC, American Psychiatric Publishing, 2003a

Paris J: Personality disorders over time: precursors, course and outcome. J Pers Disord 17(6):479–488, 2003b

Paris J: The nature of borderline personality disorder: multiple dimensions, multiple symptoms, but one category. J Pers Disord 21(5):457–473, 2007

Paton C, Crawford MJ, Bhatti SF, et al: The use of psychotropic medication in patients with emotionally unstable personality disorder under the care of UK mental health services. J Clin Psychiatry 76(4):e512–e518, 2015

Piaget J: The Psychology of Intelligence. Totowa, NJ, Littlefield, 1972

Posner MI, Rothbart MK, Vizueta N, et al: An approach to the psychobiology of personality disorders. Dev Psychopathol 15(4):1093–1106, 2003

Powers A, Casey BJ: The adolescent brain and the emergence and peak of psychopathology. Journal of Infant, Child, and Adolescent Psychotherapy 14(1):3–15, 2015

Putnam KM, Silk KR: Emotion dysregulation and the development of borderline personality disorder. Dev Psychopathol 17(4):899–925, 2005

Reyna VF: How people make decisions that involve risk: a dual-processes approach. Current Directions in Psychological Science 13(2):60–66, 2004

Reyna VF, Farley F: Risk and rationality in adolescent decision making: implications for theory, practice, and public policy. Psychol Sci Public Interest 7(1):1–44, 2006

Rogosch FA, Cicchetti D: Child maltreatment, attention networks, and potential precursors to borderline personality disorder. Dev Psychopathol 17(4):1071–1089, 2005

Romer D, Reyna VF, Satterthwaite TD: Beyond stereotypes of adolescent risk taking: placing the adolescent brain in developmental context. Dev Cog Neurosci 27:19–34, 2017

Rudolph KD: Puberty as a developmental context of risk for psychopathology, in Handbook of Developmental Psychopathology. Edited by Lewis M, Rudolph KD. New York, Springer, 2014, pp 331–354

Russell RL, Shirk SR: Child psychotherapy process research. Advances in Clinical Child Psychology 20:93–124, 1998

Sadikaj G, Russell JJ, Moskowitz DS, et al: Affect dysregulation in individuals with borderline personality disorder: persistence and interpersonal triggers. J Pers Assess 92(6):490–500, 2010

Sansone RA, Hahn HS, Dittoe N, et al: The relationship between childhood trauma and borderline personality symptomatology in a consecutive sample of cardiac stress test patients. Int J Psychiatry Clin Pract 15(4):275–279, 2011

Schneider SL, Caffray CM: Affective motivators and experience in adolescents' development of health-related behavior patterns, in The Adolescent Brain: Learning, Reasoning, and Decision Making. Edited by Reyna VF, Chapman SB, Dougherty MR, et al. Washington, DC, American Psychological Association, 2012, pp 291–335

Schwartz SJ, Beyers W, Luyckx K, et al: Examining the light and dark sides of emerging adults' identity: a study of identity status differences in positive and negative psychosocial functioning. J Youth Adolesc 40(7):839–859, 2011

Scott LN, Levy KN, Adams RB Jr, Stevenson MT: Mental state decoding abilities in young adults with borderline personality disorder traits. Personal Disord 2(2):98–112, 2011

Segal H: Introduction to the Work of Melanie Klein. New York, Basic Books, 1964

Selzer MA, Kernberg P, Fibel B, et al: The Personality Assessment Interview: preliminary report. Psychiatry 50(2):142–153, 1987

Sharp C: Current trends in BPD research as indicative of a broader sea-change in psychiatric nosology. Personal Disord 7(4):334–343, 2016

Sharp C, Fonagy P: Practitioner review: borderline personality disorder in adolescence—recent conceptualization, intervention, and implications for clinical practice. J Child Psychol Psychiatry 56(12):1266–1288, 2015

Sharp C, Wall K: Personality pathology grows up: adolescence as a sensitive period. Curr Opin Psychol 21:111–116, 2018

Sharp C, Wright AGC, Fowler JC, et al: The structure of personality pathology: both general ('g') and specific ('s') factors? J Abnorm Psychol 124(2):387–398, 2015

Shiner RL: A developmental perspective on personality disorders: lessons from research on normal personality development in childhood and adolescence. J Pers Disord 19(2):202–210, 2005

Shiner RL: The development of personality disorders: perspectives from normal personality development in childhood and adolescence. Dev Psychopathol 21(3):715–734, 2009

Shiner RL, Allen TA: Assessing personality disorders in adolescents: seven guiding principles. Clin Psychol (New York) 20(4):361–377, 2013

Shirk SR: Causal reasoning and children's comprehension of therapeutic interpretations, in Cognitive Development and Child Psychotherapy. Edited by Shirk SR. New York, Springer, 1988, pp 53–89

Silk JS, Siegle GJ, Whalen DJ, et al: Pubertal changes in emotional information processing: pupillary, behavioral, and subjective evidence during emotional word identification. Dev Psychopathol 21(1):7–26, 2009

Skodol AE: Impact of personality pathology on psychosocial functioning. Curr Opin Psychol 21:33–38, 2018

Skodol AE, Bender DS, Oldham JM: An alternative model for personality disorders: DSM-5 section III and beyond, in The American Psychiatric Publishing Textbook of Personality Disorders, 2nd Edition. Edited by Oldham JM, Skodol AE, Bender DS. Washington, DC, American Psychiatric Publishing, 2014, pp 511–544

Speranza M, Revah-Levy A, Cortese S, et al: ADHD in adolescents with borderline personality disorder. BMC Psychiatry 11(1):158, 2011

Stanovich KE, West RF: Individual differences in reasoning: implications for the rationality debate? Behav Brain Sci 23(5):645–665, 2000

Steinberg L: A social neuroscience perspective on adolescent risk-taking. Dev Rev 28(1):78–106, 2008

Stern BL, Caligor E, Hörz-Sagstetter S, et al: An object-relations based model for the assessment of borderline psychopathology. Psychiatr Clin North Am 41:595–611, 2018

Stern DN: The Motherhood Constellation: A Unified View of Parent-Infant Psychotherapy. New York, Basic Books, 1995

Tackett JL, Balsis S, Oltmanns TF, et al: A unifying perspective on personality pathology across the life span: developmental considerations for the fifth edition of the Diagnostic and Statistical Manual of Mental Disorders. Dev Psychopathol 21(3):687–713, 2009

Terr LC, Kerrnberg PF: Resolved: borderline personality exists in children under twelve. J Am Acad Child Adolesc Psychiatry 29(3):478–483, 1990

Torgersen S, Lygren S, Øien PA, et al: A twin study of personality disorders. Compr Psychiatry 41(6):416–425, 2000

Weiner AS: Theme centered group psychotherapy with psychiatrically hospitalized preadolescent boys. Group 7(1):27–33, 1983

Weiner B: Social Motivation, Justice, and the Moral Emotions: An Attributional Approach. Mahwah, NJ, Erlbaum, 2006

Westen D, Shedler J, Durrett C, et al: Personality diagnoses in adolescence: DSM-IV Axis II diagnoses and an empirically derived alternative. Am J Psychiatry 160(5):952–966, 2003

Westen D, Betan E, DeFife JA: Identity disturbance in adolescence: associations with borderline personality disorder. Dev Psychopathol 23(1):305–313, 2011

Westen D, DeFife JA, Malone JC, et al: An empirically derived classification of adolescent personality disorders. J Am Acad Child Adolesc Psychiatry 53(5):528–549, 2014

Widom CS, Czaja SJ, Paris J: A prospective investigation of borderline personality disorder in abused and neglected children followed up into adulthood. J Pers Disord 23(5):433–446, 2009

Wilcox HC, Arria AM, Caldeira KM, et al: Longitudinal predictors of past-year non-suicidal self-injury and motives among college students. Psychol Med 42(4):717–726, 2012

Winnicott C, Shepherd R, Davis M (eds): D. W. Winnicott: Deprivation and Delinquency. London, Tavistock, 1984

Winnicott DW: The antisocial tendency (1962), in The Maturational Processes and the Facilitating Environment. London, Hogarth Press/Institute of Psycho-Analysis, 1965

Winnicott DW: Playing and Reality. New York, Basic Books, 1971

Winograd G, Cohen P, Chen H: Adolescent borderline symptoms in the community: prognosis for functioning over 20 years. J Child Psychol Psychiatry 49(9):933–941, 2008

Winsper C, Marwaha S, Lereya ST, et al: Clinical and psychosocial outcomes of borderline personality disorder in childhood and adolescence: a systematic review. Psychol Med 45(11):2237–2251, 2015

World Health Organization: Guideline Development Group. Geneva, Switzerland, WHO Press, 2009

Yen S, Weinstock LM, Andover MS, et al: Prospective predictors of adolescent suicidality: 6-month post-hospitalization follow-up. Psychol Med 43:983–993, 2013

Yeomans FE, Selzer MA, Clarkin JF: Treating the Borderline Patient: A Contract-Based Approach. New York, Basic Books, 1992

Yeomans FE, Clarkin JF, Kernberg OF: Transference-Focused Psychotherapy for Borderline Personality Disorder: A Clinical Guide. Arlington, VA, American Psychiatric Publishing, 2015

Yeomans FE, Delaney JC, Levy KN: Behavioral activation in TFP: the role of the treatment contract in transference-focused psychotherapy. Psychotherapy 54(3):260–266, 2017

Zanarini MC, Frankenburg FR: The essential nature of borderline psychopathology. J Pers Disord 21(5):518–535, 2007

Zanarini MC, Williams AA, Lewis RE, et al: Reported pathological childhood experiences associated with the development of borderline personality disorder. Am J Psychiatry 154(8):1101–1106, 1997

Zanarini MC, Frankenburg FR, Reich DB, et al: Biparental failure in the childhood experiences of borderline patients. J Pers Disord 14(3):264–273, 2000

Zanarini MC, Frankenburg FR, Khera GS, et al: Treatment histories of borderline inpatients. Compr Psychiatry 42(2):144–150, 2001

Zanarini MC, Frankenburg FR, Hennen J, et al: The McLean Study of Adult Development (MSAD): overview and implications of the first six years of prospective follow-up. J Pers Disord 19(5):505–523, 2005

Zanarini MC, Frankenburg FR, Hennen J, et al: Prediction of the 10-year course of borderline personality disorder. Am J Psychiatry 163(5):827–832, 2006

Zelkowitz P, Paris J, Guzder J, et al: Diatheses and stressors in borderline pathology of childhood: the role of neuropsychological risk and trauma. J Am Acad Child Adolesc Psychiatry 40(1):100–105, 2001

# Index

Page numbers printed in **boldface** type refer to tables or figures.